sci ℷ

D0516919

FEB 2 2 1999

25ₓ (99-047)7/04
24ₓ (99-02)1/03
34 ₓ (6/07)11/07

the whole
soy cookbook

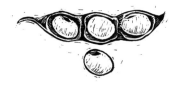

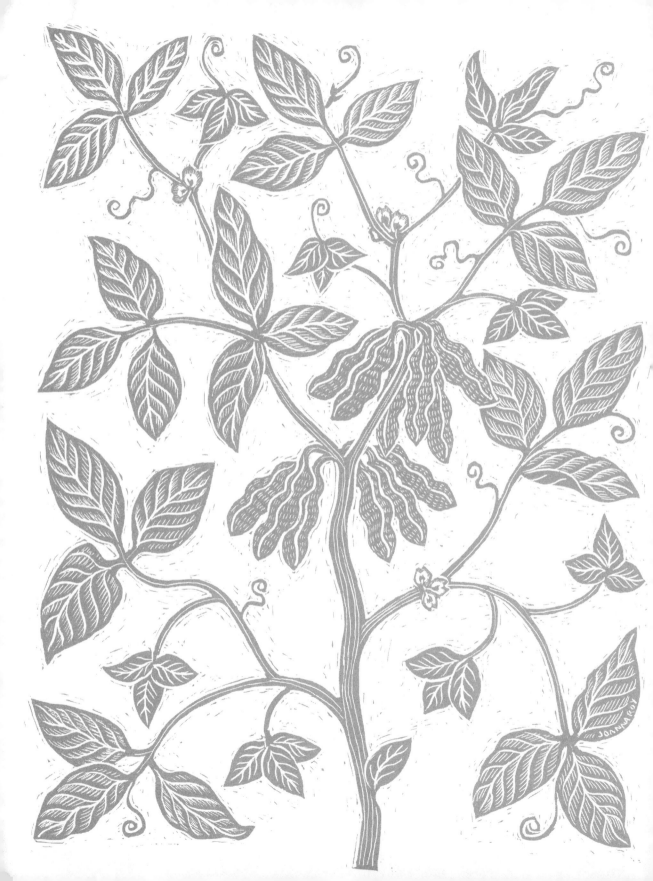

the whole
soy cookbook

175 Delicious, Nutritious, Easy-to-Prepare Recipes

Featuring Tofu, Tempeh,

and Various Forms of Nature's Healthiest Bean

PATRICIA GREENBERG

with

HELEN NEWTON HARTUNG

3 1336 04706 0356

Three Rivers Press

NEW YORK

Copyright © 1998 by Patricia Greenberg

All rights reserved. No part of this book may be reproduced or transmitted in any form or by any means, electronic or mechanical, including photocopying, recording, or by any information storage and retrieval system, without permission in writing from the publisher.

Published by Three Rivers Press, a division of Crown Publishers, Inc., 201 East 50th Street, New York, New York 10022. Member of the Crown Publishing Group.

Random House, Inc. New York, Toronto, London, Sydney, Auckland

http://www.randomhouse.com/

THREE RIVERS PRESS and colophon are trademarks of Crown Publishers, Inc.

Printed in the United States of America

DESIGN BY LYNNE AMFT

Library of Congress Cataloging-in-Publication Data

Greenberg, Patricia

The whole soy cookbook: 175 delicious, nutritious, easy-to-prepare recipes featuring tofu, tempeh, and various forms of nature's healthiest bean / by Patricia Greenberg with Helen Newton Hartung.

1. Cookery (Soybeans).   2. Soyfoods—Therapeutic use.   I. Hartung, Helen Newton.   II. Title.

TX803.S6G74   1998

641.6'5655—dc21   97–19011

ISBN 0-517-88813-0

10 9 8 7 6 5 4 3 2 1

First Edition

This book is dedicated to my parents,
Joan and David Greenberg,
and my siblings,
Elizabeth, Bert, Stephen, and Janice,
who have given me unconditional love
and support my whole life
and have always helped me
move forward.

contents

acknowledgments

Writing a cookbook is an arduous project that requires a team of dedicated people to bring it to fruition. To make *The Whole Soy Cookbook* a reality, I called upon many people for help and they all came through for me in a variety of ways.

First and foremost I want to thank my coauthor, Helen Newton Hartung. Her creativity, excellent writing skills, and vast knowledge of food made the recipes and information come alive on paper. This book would not have happened without her.

I am overflowing with gratitude for my agent, Betsy Amster. She believed in my idea and provided me with the opportunity to present my work to Crown Publishers. Guiding me as a first-time author, she held my hand through the whole process to a successful completion.

It is with tremendous respect and admiration that I would like to thank my editors at Crown: Wendy Hubbert, who kept the focus on the big picture every step of the way, and PJ Dempsey, for her creativity and amazing ability to pull it all together for me.

I would also like to acknowledge David Mintz, of Tofutti Foods, and Tom McReynolds, of Mori-Nu Tofu, for supplying me with lots of encouragement, insight into the soyfood industry, and tons of delicious soy products for recipe development.

I wish to thank all my dear friends for encouraging me and giving me honest feedback on several of my soy recipes. And I especially want to thank Aaron A. Grunfeld whose love and support kept me going through some very frustrating times. He started out as a skeptic, and is now a firm believer in the miracles of soy.

the whole
soy cookbook

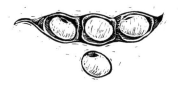

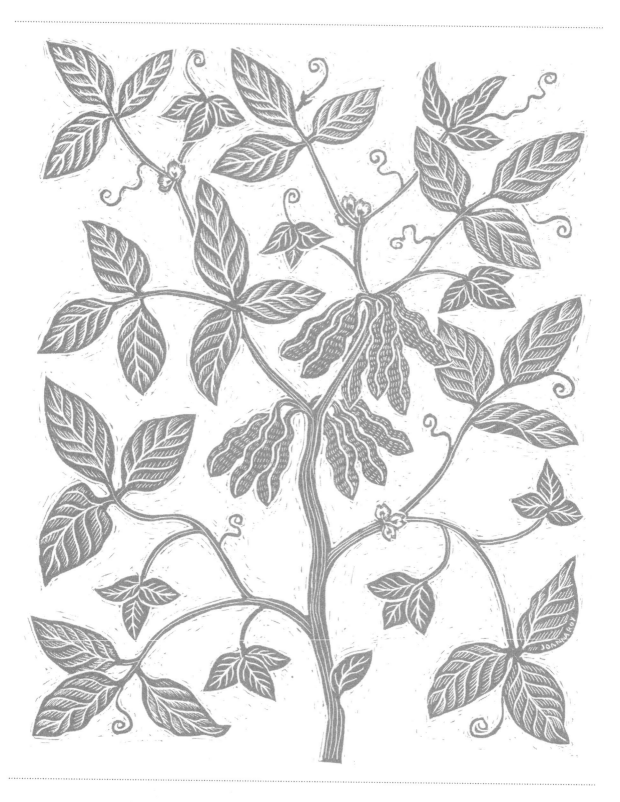

introduction

Imagine you had the power to create the perfect food, a substance so wonderful it could solve many of the world's nutritional ills. What would it be like?

First of all, it would have to be delicious. It would have to be easy to work with and so versatile that it would never become boring. It would have to provide inexpensive and complete nutrition. It would have no cholesterol and no saturated fat and so would cause no ill effects to the human body. Even better, it would actually help prevent—perhaps even reverse—some of the world's most dreaded diseases. It would be easy and cheap to produce and it could be grown in a variety of soils and climates. Its cultivation wouldn't deplete the earth of nutrients and would even enhance the environment.

The fact is, we don't need to imagine this "miracle food" because it already exists. It is called soy.

If you are picking up this book, you have probably heard some of the recent medical news about soy's miraculous health properties—how eating as little as 25 grams of soy protein a day can prevent heart disease, breast cancer, and prostate cancer, among other illnesses. Or perhaps you are already familiar with soy and seek new and exciting ways of cooking healthfully for your family. Whether you're an experienced vegetarian cook or a newcomer to health-conscious cooking, this unique cookbook is for you. Its purpose is to make it easy—as well as delicious—for anyone to gain the benefits of including soy in his or her diet.

Who benefits from soy? The list is long: anyone concerned about preventing heart disease; anyone interested in preventing breast cancer; anyone with worries about prostate cancer or colon cancer; anyone with milk allergies or lactose intolerance, including infants who can't digest regular baby formulas; women anxious to ease the symptoms of menopause; anyone who suffers from digestive problems or diabetes. Everyone, in fact, can benefit from soy, since soy provides high-quality, inexpensive protein chock-full of vitamins, minerals, and fiber but with absolutely no cholesterol or saturated fat. But most important of all, soy—and only soy—contains a compound called *genistein,* which has been scientifically proven in many major studies to possess remarkable powers of healing and prevention. Adding soy protein to your diet makes sense for everyone.

This book contains almost 200 delicious and easy ways for you to add that essential 25 grams of soy protein to your diet. In over ten years of experimenting, refining, cooking for friends, and teaching others, I have created a wealth of exciting soy-based recipes, many inspired by classics from the world's best cuisines. The recipes in this book do not use any meat, eggs, or dairy products—be sure to check the labels of soy products because a few of them contain trace amounts of milk protein—making them perfect for vegans, the strict vegetarians who eliminate all animal products from their diets, and the lactose intolerant, who cannot digest milk.

Lacto-vegetarians—those who eat vegetables, grains, and dairy products—can benefit from this book, too. You can continue to use regular dairy products if you wish, substituting equal amounts in those recipes here calling for soy milk and soy cheese. You'll still receive plenty of the healthy benefits of soy by choosing recipes featuring tofu, tempeh, and meat analogs. Keep in mind, however, that soy milks, soy cheeses, and soy-based egg replacers serve exactly the same functions as their dairy counterparts, providing high protein, calcium, vitamins, and great flavor, but without any saturated fat or cholesterol. And only soy products provide genistein.

Even if you don't consider yourself a vegetarian, you are probably trying to follow FDA nutritional guidelines by reducing your intake of meats and fats while emphasizing fruits, vegetables, and grains. Like many people, you may have eliminated red meats in favor of occasional, small servings of lean chicken and fish. I think of this growing category as semi-vegetarians. Semi-vegetarians will find this book a blessing, too. It will introduce you to a new range of healthy, protein-packed food choices. Because soy products come in a variety of mouthwatering forms that can be cooked and seasoned just like many meats (learn more about these products beginning on page 10), semi-vegetarians will miss nothing and gain much by including soy in their diets.

Whether you're vegan, vegetarian, or semi-vegetarian, you will find wonderful taste treats here. There's a spicy South of the Border Tofu Salad (page 61), a summery grilled Garden Kabob (page 155), crowd-pleasing Soybean

Chili (page 134), and Soy Cheese Pizza (page 110), plus satisfying Whole Wheat Banana Soy Muffins (page 95), Soy Sour Cream Lemon Loaf (page 101), and dazzling desserts such as creamy Tofu Chocolate Mousse (page 191)—all made with soy. You'll find hearty stews and velvety "cream" soups; down-home meat loaf and uptown crepes. Whatever you can imagine making with other foods and any cuisine—from elegant French cooking to comfortable American, hot-blooded Mexican to full-flavored Chinese—I have adapted a recipe using the wealth of soy products.

You may be completely new to the world of soy products or you may be familiar with some forms of soy but not with others. This book will be your guide. It contains innovative recipes featuring such soy products as smooth and versatile tofu, firm and nutty tempeh cakes, creamy soy milk, delicious soy cheeses, and amazingly realistic and nutritious soy "meats." In the "Cooking with Soy" section of this Introduction, you'll find a complete guide to these products, with information on what they are, where to buy them, and how to cook and store them. You'll want to experiment with all these forms of the miraculous bean to find which you most enjoy and which you feel most comfortable working with.

Every recipe includes a nutritional analysis, so it's easy to see just how many grams of soy protein a given dish provides. On page 27, there's a sample analysis to get you started. Following that you'll find a week's worth of sample menus that demonstrate just how effortless it is to add at least 25 grams of soy protein a day to your diet.

all about soy

If you've read this far, you have some general knowledge about the amazing benefits of including soy protein in your diet. To find out more specifically how using the recipes in this book can benefit your health, let's look at the evidence.

health benefits of soy

Soy reduces the risk of heart disease: It is a fact that the occurrence of heart disease is substantially lower in Japan than in America. Why? Scientists believe that the high soy content—specifically the high genistein content—in the Japanese diet makes the difference. For example, a recent study reported in the *New England Journal of Medicine* stated that participants who consumed 17 to 25 grams of soy protein a day reduced their serum cholesterol 9.3 percent on average. Furthermore, their levels of low-density lipoprotein cholesterol (LDL, or "bad cholesterol") declined 13 percent, while levels of "good cholesterol," or HDL, were unaffected. Soy also contains an essential oil, linoleic acid, which is one of the Omega-3 fatty acids linked to the reduction of heart disease. Study participants with the highest levels of cholesterol showed the greatest improvement, as did those who consumed the greatest amounts of soy. The conclusion reached in the *New England Journal of Medicine* study was that regular intake of soy protein could reduce the risk of heart disease by 20 to 30 percent. That's a remarkable statistic: simply by eating 25 grams of soy protein a day, you can reduce by almost one-third your chances of falling prey to our country's number-one killer, heart disease.

Soy lowers the risk of breast cancer: Breast cancer rates in Asian countries are four to five times lower than in the United States. Here, too, scientists believe soy protein and genistein deserve the credit. In some studies, researchers have demonstrated that genistein can block the formation of breast cancer cells.

Since 1994, scientists at premier medical and research institutions have published more than 250 studies and papers on this promising soy-based approach to combating breast cancer.

In one such study, performed at the University of Alabama, laboratory animals were injected with substances that cause breast cancer. Some animals were then fed a standard diet while others were fed a diet high in soybeans. Those fed the soybean diet developed fewer tumors. Scientists explain it this way: genistein is similar in structure to estrogen, though much weaker. Genistein and other substances found in soybeans are known as phytoestrogens, which means "plant-based estrogens." When a woman consumes soy foods, these phytoestrogens fill the estrogen receptor sites in breast tissue, making it impossible for excess human estrogen to bind in those tissues and cause destructive changes. Eating merely 25 grams of soy protein a day seems to be enough to help prevent breast cancer.

Soy eases the symptoms of menopause: You can reduce the unpleasant symptoms of menopause—such as hot flashes, mood swings, and excess hair growth—simply by eating soy foods. The same genistein that helps prevent breast cancer by blocking estrogen's ability to cause malignant changes can help here, too. During menopause, a woman's body significantly reduces its production of estrogen. This loss of estrogen causes classic menopausal symptoms. Genistein and other phytoestrogens from soy make the body think it is receiving estrogen (though in a weaker, safer form) by filling the estrogen receptors. One cup of soybeans or a soy product such as tofu or soy milk produces as much estrogen activity as a 0.45 milligram Premarin tablet—a commonly prescribed medication for the symptoms of menopause—without the increased cancer risk associated with estrogen therapy.

Soy protects against prostate cancer: According to a study performed at the University of Alabama, the genistein found only in soy foods may inhibit the growth of prostate cancer cells. Scientists have concluded that a low rate of prostate cancer among Japanese men is directly related to the high levels of genistein found in their diets. A study currently underway at the University of California at Los Angeles aims to substantiate this theory. In the study, men with high prostate specific antigen levels (indicative of inflammation or the presence of cancer cells in the prostate) are eating a low-fat, high-soy diet to determine exactly how effective genistein is in reducing the growth of those localized cancer cells.

Soy prevents digestive disorders: Diverticulitis is an intensely painful medical condition caused by pockets of infection in the colon. Constipation and hemorrhoids can also be serious problems for many people. Increasing the amount of soy in your diet can prevent or substantially lessen the effects of all three of these problems. Soybeans and many soy products contain high levels of fiber (6 grams of fiber per cup of cooked soybeans), which cleanses the colon as it passes through and prevents painful diverticulitis pockets from forming. Fiber promotes bowel movement regularity, which helps prevent both constipation and hemorrhoids. Studies also show that people who consume a high-fiber diet have substantially lower colon and rectal cancer rates.

Soy eliminates the problem of lactose intolerance: Milk, infant formula, and cheese made from soy are an obvious solution for babies and adults who suffer the often painful condition of lactose intolerance. These individuals cannot digest dairy milk or milk products because their systems lack the digestive enzyme lactase, needed to break down milk sugar into usable energy and nutrients. The usual symptoms of this condition are bloating and swelling of the intestines, diarrhea, and, in severe cases, nausea. Although some infants are afflicted with lactose intolerance, the condition is more common among adults and seems to increase with age. As we grow older, we tend to drink less milk and thus our bodies produce less lactase, which in turn leads to lactose intolerance. People of African, Asian, and Middle Eastern origins are most likely to suffer from this condition. Using the delicious soy recipes in this book will allow anyone with lactose intolerance to enjoy lactose-free versions of such previously off-limits foods as pizza, rich cream soups, and mouthwatering cheesecakes.

Soy prevents the problems of milk allergy: Many people have allergic reactions to certain foods, one of the most common of which is dairy milk. Soy milk products, on the other hand, have a very low rate of associated allergic reactions. Allergies occur when the body perceives a food molecule as a foreign, and possibly harmful, substance and develops antibodies to fight it. Once the antibodies form, the body will always reject that type of food. Symptoms of milk allergy are similar to those of lactose intolerance, although milk allergy may also give rise to rashes and other forms of skin irritation. Infants, in particular, are highly susceptible to milk allergies, which is why wholesome soy baby formulas are so popular among parents and health professionals. As with lactose intolerance, if you have milk allergies you have had to give up many favorite foods, from pizza to ice cream. Not any longer, thanks to the recipes in this book, which substitute soy milk and cheese for dairy products. Soy milk and baby formulas provide protein and calcium levels comparable to those of dairy milk.

Soy is beneficial in diabetic diets: Scientists believe there are several ways in which soy foods can help diabetics, who suffer from an inability to control blood sugar levels. Since soybeans do not cause the body's blood sugar levels to rise very much (such foods are said therefore to have a low glycemic index), when eating soy products a diabetic may be less concerned about unhealthy fluctuations. Also, because soybeans are high in fiber, they help slow the body's absorption of nutrients, which helps keep a diabetic's blood sugar levels on an even keel. Diabetics are more susceptible than others to heart disease, and because soy protein has been shown to reduce levels of cholesterol, it can help prevent this common—and deadly—complication.

Clearly, adding soy protein to your diet has many remarkable benefits. At this point, however, you may be wondering: What exactly *are* soy foods? What forms are best to cook with? How do I know how much to eat? Does sprinkling soy sauce on my Chinese food count? I'll answer those questions and more, starting from the ground up, with a little background on the soybean itself.

The scientific name of the soybean is *Glycine max,* and it is a member of the legume family. The soy plant grows about two feet tall. It has a woody stem with broad leaves, flowers, and seed pods, the latter which house the beans themselves. As a soybean plant develops, the leaves, stems, and growing pods are covered with soft brownish-green hairs. The seed pods are 1½ to 2 inches long, and each pod contains two to three beans. Soybeans that are grown in Asia tend to be larger than their American and Canadian counterparts.

The word *soy* has both Chinese and Japanese origins. The ancient Chinese, who first documented the use of soybeans in the fifteenth century B.C., called them *sou*. Present-day Chinese call soybeans *ta-tou,* which means "great beans." The Japanese call soy sauce *shoyu.* Our term soy could have come from either of these sources. Ironically, the United States is by far the largest producer of soybeans in the world, but Americans consume relatively few of them in their daily diets. Most of the soybeans grown in this country are processed into soy oil, used widely in vegetable oils, shortenings and margarines, and high-protein animal feed. The Japanese, in contrast, consume twice as much soy protein per person, yet produce very little.

The cultivation of soybeans, unlike that of most agricultural crops, actually improves the soil in which they are grown. Most cropland needs to be rotated, or planted with different crops, every few years so the land can lie fallow and restore its fertility. A soybean crop, however, keeps the soil rich in nutrients and can be grown over and over again without rotation. In fact, when the plant was first introduced to this country, it was called "green manure" because of its positive effect on the soil.

Fresh soybeans are similar in size and color to green peas. They are harvested in early July, when the pods are still immature, and are sold while they are still green. The rest of the soy crop is harvested in late September or early October, when the leaves have fallen from the plants and the mature beans have dried on the vine. Dried beans are usually yellow-beige, although there are green, purple, brown, black, and even spotted varieties. Dried beans are sold in bulk to farmers, ranchers, and food manufacturers for a wide variety of uses.

Of all legumes, soybeans have the highest concentration of protein: most other beans contain 20 percent protein by volume, while soybeans have 40 percent. Soy products are cholesterol free and high in calcium, phosphorous, and fiber. Soy consumed in its original form is able to provide an enormous amount of raw protein in the human diet. A beef cow, fed about 18 pounds of vegetable protein, will yield only 1 pound of protein from meat. Getting protein from the soybean and other plant sources is therefore not only good for us but good for the environment, too.

Once you start cooking with soy, you'll wonder how you ever lived without it. You'll feel better, mentally and physically; you will be consuming health-giving levels of genistein while simultaneously eliminating major sources of fat and cholesterol. Soy products are easy to find and buy, easy to store, and a cinch to cook with, performing almost exactly like dairy milk and cheese and animal meats.

Best of all, soy foods are unbelievably delicious, as you'll see when you whip up some of the fabulous foods in this book. As you delight in creamy Soy Fettuccine Alfredo (page 168) or spicy Tempeh Fajitas (page 152); as you devour Chocolate Soy Brownies (page 188) or Peaches and Cream Brûlée (page 202), you'll be thrilled to discover what is truly a miracle food. Welcome to *The Whole Soy Cookbook*!

cooking with soy products

Because more and more people are becoming aware of the benefits of eating soy, food manufacturers are rapidly creating new soy products. In the past decade, as many as 2,000 new items have found their way into our stores. Consider the wealth of existing products such as tofu, soy milk, and tempeh, and it's easy to become confused. Which should you add to your diet and how? Let's start at the beginning. Here is a list of the major types of foods that come from the soybean.

Meat analogs or meat substitutes	Soybeans, whole, roasted (also known as soy nuts) and green
Miso	
Okara	Tempeh
Soy cheese	Tofu
Soy flour	Egg replacers
Soy milk	Soy margarine
Soy sour cream	Soy mayonnaise
Soy yogurt	Soy sauce
Textured vegetable protein (TVP)	Soybean oil

Some of these soy products may be familiar to you while others may seem exotic and perplexing. But either way, you'll find it easy to incorporate many of these products into everyday meal planning. That being said, note that it is neither practical nor necessary to cook with all of these products all the time. In fact, a few of these foods—such as okara—are not very useful in the home kitchen, though I have listed it in the interest of thoroughness.

Looking at this list of foods, you may have many questions: can you cook dried soybeans like any other dried legume? How long does soy milk keep? Does soy cheese melt like dairy cheese? How is tofu stored? Let's take a closer look at these foods so you can learn exactly what the various types of soy foods are, where to find them, which ones are most practical for home use, and how to store and use them. I have mentioned brand names of some products to make it easier for you to look for them; I have also provided a complete list of soy suppliers on pages 211 and 212. I will also show you which soy foods to look for to get the highest amounts of beneficial genistein and soy protein.

Meat Analogs or Meat Substitutes

This category of foods consists of soy-based products that simulate different meats and meat products. Meat analogs, such as soy bacon, soy ham, soy sausage, soy hot dogs, and soy hamburgers, are made primarily from textured vegetable protein (TVP) and soy protein concentrate. They are an excellent source of protein, vitamin B_{12}, and iron. Soy meat analogs also contain high levels of genistein. The fat content varies, though all soy meats are substantially lower in fat and calories than real meat.

Some of the easy-to-use meat analogs are:

Soy sausage: You can find formed soy sausage links in a variety of styles—breakfast, chorizo, Cajun, Italian, and smoked. You can also find preformed patties in various sizes and flavors. Ground soy sausage makes a wonderful substitute for ground beef or pork and it is available retail in 14-ounce plastic tube packages just like traditional pork sausage. Morningstar Farms and Lite Life's Gimme Lean are two readily available brands of formed sausages and ground soy sausage. Green Giant manufactures links and patties. Green Giant and Morningstar Farms' products can be found in grocery stores, while Lite Life's products are generally carried in health food stores and specialty markets. Experiment with the various brands to see which you prefer.

Use preformed link sausages in recipes such as Soy Sausage Paella (page 162) or Cajun Red Hot Jambalaya with Soy Sausage (page 164), in which the sausage must keep its shape. Or serve cooked link sausage or patty sausage just as you would traditional sausage—as part of a hearty breakfast or brunch, along with fruit and hot cereal or Whole Wheat Banana Soy Muffins (page 95), for example. Ground soy sausage is even more versatile. Use it as you would ground beef, ground turkey, or sausage meat: in meat loaves, pizza toppings, meat sauces, and casseroles. All forms of soy sausage are very low in fat; you will obtain best results if you brown them in nonstick pans coated with a little vegetable oil spray or soybean oil. Stir frequently to prevent sticking. Soy sausages must be kept refrigerated and should be consumed within two weeks of being opened.

Soy bacon: This product is made from soy protein isolates or tempeh. It contains genistein and provides all the other benefits of soy in addition to being fat free. Soy bacon comes in two forms: bacon bits and bacon strips. The bacon bits, precooked and packaged in a plastic container, have been around for a long time and are widely available in supermarkets. There are two types of bacon strips, both of which resemble real bacon strips, made by Morningstar Farms and Lite Life. Packaged like real bacon, they are available in the freezer or refrigerator case. Grocery stores carry Morningstar Farms bacon, while health food stores are the source for the Lite Life brand.

Use soy bacon bits to top salads or baked potatoes. They keep indefinitely on the pantry shelf. Soy bacon strips can be used in all the many ways you would use regular bacon. They cook very quickly—one minute per side—and tend to stick to the pan because they have no fat. Use nonstick pans coated with a little cooking spray. The strips must be refrigerated and consumed within two weeks of opening.

Hamburgers and hot dogs: Some of the many hamburgers and hot dogs on the market these days are made of only soy protein isolates, while others have grains and vegetables added. All of these meat analogs are excellent sources of soy protein and genistein.

Soy hamburgers come preformed into patties. Morningstar Farms, Green Giant, and Yves are just a few of the brands available in supermarkets and health food stores. In supermarkets, look for these products in the frozen food department, while health food stores may sell fresh versions as well. Experiment among the various brands to find the ones you and your family like best. Hot dogs manufactured by Lite Life and Soy Boy, among others, some-times contain tofu as well as soy protein isolates. Look for these products in grocery and health food stores.

Use these products just as you would real hot dogs and hamburgers. Cook them on the grill, in the broiler, or on the stovetop and serve them with or with-out buns. The only difference between preparing soy hot dogs or hamburgers and the originals is that the soy products cook more quickly. Spray the grill or pan with cooking spray or use nonstick pans, as these low-fat products other-wise tend to stick to the pan. Refrigerate soy hot dogs and soy hamburger prod-ucts and consume them within one week of opening the packages.

Soy Meat Versus Animal Meat (3-ounce portions)

Item	Calories	Protein (grams)	Carb. (grams)	Fat (grams)	Chol. (mg)	Fiber (grams)	Sodium (mg)
Ground beef	171	14	0	12	51	0	36
Ground soy	105	14	100	0	0	1	290
Pork sausage links	314	16	0	26	70	0	1099
Soy sausage links	120	10	5	4	0	0	160
Pork bacon	490	26	0.5	15	72	0	1364
Soy bacon	80	8	6	2.5	0	0	230

MISO

Made from fermented soybeans, miso is a salty paste of Japanese origin. Miso contains 12 to 21 percent protein, comparable to chicken (20 percent), and substantial quantities of genistein. It is high in B vitamins but also in sodium.

You can buy 8-ounce plastic tubs of miso from Asian markets and health food stores. With a texture like soft peanut butter, it comes in a range of colors and flavors. It may be strong, mild, red, yellow, or white; made only of soy-beans or of soybeans combined with grains.

Miso is most widely used as a soup base (I include a light, Japanese-inspired miso soup in this book on page 120), but it can also be used as a condiment and added for taste to stews, sauces, marinades, and dressings. Because it is a fermented food, it keeps for a long time, unrefrigerated.

OKARA

After soybeans are pressed to make soy milk, the flaky pulp that remains becomes okara. It is a good source of protein and fiber. However, because okara is not readily available to consumers in the United States, I do not include recipes for it here. It is used commercially in manufacturing meat analogs and some baked goods.

SOY CHEESE

Just as dairy milk is processed into various kinds of cheeses, soy milk can be made into similar products. Although soy cheese closely resembles regular cheese in texture and usage, it is cholesterol free and lower in fat than its dairy counterpart. There is a trace of milk protein in some soy cheeses, so those who wish to avoid all dairy products should be sure to check the labels carefully. Vegan varieties are available.

Soy cheese comes in full-fat, low-fat, and nonfat versions. Firm cheeses, such as mozzarella, jack, and cheddar, come in 8- to 12-ounce packages, rather like dairy cheese. Soya-Kaas, Soy Sensation, and Soymage are three widely distributed brands that you can find in supermarkets or health food stores, in or near the dairy section.

Soy parmesan cheese is indistinguishable from regular grated parmesan; however, soy parmesan comes only pregrated, not in chunks or wheels. It contains 2 grams of soy protein per 2 teaspoons. Soy parmesan is available in both a vegan version and a variety that contains some milk fat. Soy parmesan is usually stocked only in health food stores. Soymage is one common brand.

Soy cream cheese, remarkably similar to its dairy counterpart, is cholesterol free and works well as a spread, either by itself or whipped up with other ingredients. It is sold in plastic tubs, just like whipped cream cheese, and found in grocery stores and health food stores. Some cream cheeses come in spiced versions, with herbs and garlic, pepper, or cinnamon and raisins added. Tofutti and Soya-Kaas are well-known brands. Use soy cheeses just as you would their dairy counterparts—sliced, with crackers, or cooked in recipes.

It is important to use full-fat cheeses in dishes that require cooking, such as pizzas or casseroles, because they melt better. Low-fat cheeses do not melt fluidly and are best used cool or at room temperature. In baking with soy cream cheese, use lower oven temperatures than you would with dairy cream cheese; higher temperatures could cause the cheese to separate as even full-fat soy cheese contains significantly less fat than its dairy counterpart.

Soy Milk

This creamy liquid is made by soaking and cooking whole soybeans. The beans are then ground and the milky liquid is pressed out. The milk contains no cholesterol in comparison to low-fat dairy milk, which contains 18 milligrams of cholesterol per cup. Skim milk has a trace amount of cholesterol. Soy milk is high in protein and naturally contains calcium, though more calcium is often added.

Soy milk comes in whole, low-fat, or nonfat varieties, either plain or with vanilla, chocolate, or other flavoring. It is sold in airtight, 1-quart cartons that can be stored in the pantry for up to six months. It is also the main ingredient in soy-based infant formulas, which are widely available in all types of markets. Look for soy milk in grocery stores, health food stores, and specialty markets.

Soy milk has a nutty flavor and can be used on breakfast cereal or as a substitute for dairy milk in milkshakes, cream soups, and sauces. You can choose to use regular, low-fat, or nonfat milk in almost any of these recipes, with a few exceptions. In cooked desserts, such as custards or flans, it is important to use regular or low-fat soy milk rather than nonfat because it results in a firmer consistency. Once opened, soy milk should be refrigerated and consumed within a week. You can, of course, substitute regular milk for soy milk in any of my recipes, but of course you eliminate valuable soy protein by doing so.

Soy Sour Cream

Soy sour cream is made by adding a souring agent to soy milk (the same technique used in the production of dairy sour cream). It contains no lactose or cholesterol and has about 1 gram of soy protein per serving. Soy sour cream comes in 8-ounce plastic containers. It is available in the "gourmet" cheese or kosher section of many supermarkets and in health food stores. You can use soy sour cream exactly as you would dairy sour cream, since it has the same consistency and cooking properties. It is delicious as a topping for baked potatoes or as a finishing touch for some soups. You may substitute equal quantities of soy sour cream in any recipe calling for dairy sour cream and vice versa. It should be refrigerated, where it will keep for two weeks after opening.

SOY YOGURT

Like dairy yogurt, soy yogurt is made by adding live bacteria cultures to soy milk. It is lactose and cholesterol free. One cup of soy yogurt contains 12 grams of soy protein. Soy yogurt comes in 8-ounce cups, either plain or fruit flavored, or in 16-ounce containers, in plain or vanilla flavor. It is available in health food stores in whole or low-fat varieties. You can use soy yogurt just as you would dairy yogurt: on its own as a snack or as an ingredient in soups, salad dressings, sauces, milkshakes, and desserts. Its consistency and cooking properties are identical to those of dairy yogurt. Soy yogurt keeps about a week under refrigeration.

Dairy Products Versus Soy Products

Item	Calories	Protein (grams)	Carb. (grams)	Fat (grams)	Chol. (mg)	Fiber (grams)	Sodium (mg)
Cream cheese (1 ounce)	100	2	1	10	31	0	85
Soy cream cheese (1 ounce)	80	1.5	1	8	0	0	135
Sour cream (2 tablespoons)	61	<1	1	6	13	0	15
Soy sour cream (2 tablespoons)	40	1	3	3	0	0	30
Nonfat yogurt (1 cup)	127	13	17	0.4	4	0	174
Low-fat yogurt (1 cup)	144	12	16	3.5	14	0	159
Soy yogurt (1 cup)	182	12	17	6.5	0	4	55
Mozzarella cheese (1 ounce)	72	7	1	6	16	0	132
Soy mozzarella (1 ounce)	70	6	1	5	0	0	220

Item	Calories	Protein (grams)	Carb. (grams)	Fat (grams)	Chol. (mg)	Fiber (grams)	Sodium (mg)
Whole milk (1 cup)	150	8	12	8	33	0	120
Low-fat milk (1 cup)	121	8	12	5	18	0	122
Nonfat milk (1 cup)	86	8	12	0	4	0	126
Soy milk whole (1 cup)	79	6.6	4	4.5	0	1	29
Soy milk nonfat (1 cup)	70	3	14	0	0	0	75
Parmesan cheese (2 teaspoons)	19	1	0	1	3	0	77
Soy parmesan (2 teaspoons)	15	2	1	0	0	0	85

SOY FLOUR

Soy flour is made from ground, dried soybeans and is rich in high-quality protein and other nutrients. Soy flour comes in 2-pound packages and can be hard to find, even in health food stores. Because it is more moist and dense than grain-based flours, it cannot be used by itself in baked goods. It can, however, replace up to 20 percent of the all-purpose flour called for in recipes for breads, cakes, and muffins. It is especially easy to add to recipes as you work your way through the book. Keep soy flour in the refrigerator or freezer, as it goes rancid quickly.

SOYBEANS

Whole soybeans are the simplest soy food. They look like black-eyed peas without the black eye. They are substantially higher in protein than other types of beans and are a great source of genistein. Whole soybeans are available in several forms, the most basic of which are canned and dried. Canned soybeans are precooked and come in 14-ounce cans. Dried soybeans are mature beans that have been harvested and dried. Like other dried beans, they are sold in 1-pound plastic packages. Both forms are produced by Westbrae Foods and are usually available in health food stores.

Canned soybeans are recipe ready and may be added to chilies and soups just like other canned beans. As with any dried beans, dried soybeans should be treated in the following manner: wash and soak the beans overnight in water. Drain them, cover with fresh water, and simmer the beans over low heat for three hours. They are then ready for use in recipes. Note that even when fully cooked, both dried and canned soybeans remain firmer than other beans, such as kidney or pinto. Once you realize that the slight chewiness of the beans does not mean the dish is undercooked, you can appreciate the texture soybeans add to soups, stews, and chilies. Once cooked, soybeans should be consumed within a day or two.

Soybeans Versus Other Beans (4-ounce portions, cooked)

Item	Calories	Protein (grams)	Carb. (grams)	Fat (grams)	Chol. (mg)	Fiber (grams)	Sodium (mg)
Soy beans	202	18	14	10	0	4.5	2
Navy beans	161	10	30	0	0	6	1
Pinto beans	156	9	29	0	0	3	2
Black beans	150	10	26	0	0	6	1
Lima beans	139	8	26	0	0	10	19
Lentils	132	10	22	0	0	9	3

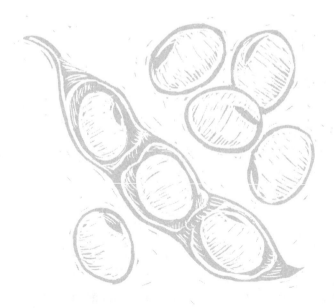

SOYBEANS, GREEN

Another form of whole soybean, fresh green soybeans are picked before they are fully mature and are usually left in their pods. They are high in protein and genistein. They resemble Chinese snow peas and are usually sold in bulk, like fresh produce, or frozen in 1-pound plastic bags. Look for green soybeans, fresh or frozen, in Asian markets or health food stores. Green soybeans make a nutritious, high-protein snack. Try serving them as an appetizer before dinner, as traditional Japanese restaurants do. Prepare by steaming for 20 minutes until slightly softened, then chill. Serve lightly salted.

SOYBEANS, ROASTED

Also known as soy nuts, roasted soybeans are a delicious, high-protein alternative to other roasted nuts. They are made by soaking whole soybeans in water, then draining and roasting them in a little oil. They are not a low-fat item, but they are high in genistein and protein (37 percent versus 26 percent for roasted peanuts). They resemble dry-roasted peanuts. Sold in 1-pound plastic bags in health food stores, they make delicious snacks or hors d'oeuvres. I also use them as a tasty high-protein addition to the Soy Nut Granola recipe on page 84. They keep at least a month and do not require refrigeration.

TEMPEH

Tempeh is made of whole, cooked soybeans that are fermented to form a dense, chewy cake. Thought to have originated in Indonesia, tempeh was originally developed as an inexpensive, high-quality meat alternative. Tempeh contains genistein, protein, and plenty of vitamin B_{12}. It is cholesterol free and contains only small amounts of fat. Its flavor is nutty and rich, though it will absorb the flavors of whatever food you combine it with. When served with grains such as rice or whole wheat, ounce-for-ounce tempeh provides the same high-quality protein as meat.

Tempeh is available in vacuum-sealed, plastic-wrapped 8-ounce patties in the refrigerator or freezer cases of health food stores and in some large grocery stores. Tempeh is firm and can be used like many forms of meat: it will maintain its shape while grilled, baked, broiled, steamed, or fried. Crumbled, it can be added like ground beef to casseroles or sauces. It can be frozen or stored in the refrigerator, where it will last about two weeks.

Textured Vegetable Protein (TVP)

Made from defatted soy flakes, TVP is a dried, granular product sold in health food stores. It may be purchased in bulk or in a 1-pound bag. It is the main ingredient of many commercially made meat substitutes such as soy sausage, soy bacon, vegetable burgers, and soy hot dogs. It is also used as a filler for processed foods.

TVP, when it first became popular about twenty years ago, was hailed as a budget-conscious way to extend ground beef. But because modern products made with TVP are easier to use and better tasting than TVP alone, I don't use TVP itself in cooking. It may be used in a pinch if you are out of soy sausage. Use an equal amount of TVP instead, reconstituting according to package directions.

Tofu

Tofu is curdled soy milk. It is made by adding nigari (a compound from sea water), calcium sulfate, and vinegar or lemon juice to soy milk. Excess moisture is squeezed out and the remaining curds are pressed into soft blocks. Also known as bean curd, tofu provides essential protein needed for human growth and maintenance. A 7-ounce serving of tofu provides 16 grams of protein: less than a comparable serving of beef (43 grams), but with no cholesterol (beef has 179 grams) and far fewer calories and fat (beef has 68 grams versus tofu's 9 grams). It comes in whole, low-fat, and nonfat varieties, and you can buy it in four forms:

1. In 12.3-ounce, aseptically sealed cartons, which can be stored unopened on pantry shelves for up to ten months. This form of tofu is available in several consistencies: soft, regular, firm, and extra-firm. Many grocery stores and all health food stores carry this product.

2. Packed in water and sealed in 1-pound plastic containers. This form comes in soft, regular, and firm consistencies and is carried by grocery stores and health food stores.

3. Fresh, sold in bulk out of open containers. I don't recommend buying tofu

in this form, as it carries a serious risk of bacterial contamination. This form is sold only in specialty or ethnic markets.

4. Freeze-dried, in small pouches. This type of tofu requires no refrigeration and has a long shelf life. To use, you must reconstitute it with boiling water. While it is handy when traveling or camping, other forms of tofu work better in most recipes. Freeze-dried tofu is available in health and camping stores.

Tofu works well in stir-fries, egglike scrambles, soups, baked goods, purees, and desserts. Most of the recipes in this book will specify which consistency of tofu—firm, soft, or silken—to use. Don't worry if you don't have the exact consistency called for. Although you will get the best results if you use the specified type, if necessary you can cook with whatever you have on hand. In general, use firm tofu as a substitute for meats in main entrees, in stir-fries, casseroles, soups, and cheesecakes. Soft tofu makes smooth dips, dressings, custards, and puddings. Use silken tofu for pureed or blended dishes. Tofu must be refrigerated after it is opened (or reconstituted, in the case of freeze-dried). You must change the water in the water-packed type every day while it is refrigerated. Once opened and refrigerated, tofu will keep about a week.

Silken tofu. This is a method of processing tofu that creates a silky smooth surface. It comes soft, regular, and firm.

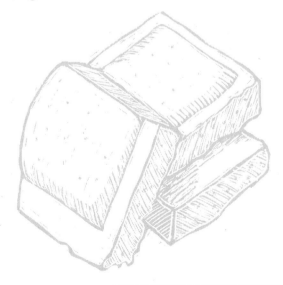

Soy Protein Versus Animal Protein (7-ounce portions)

Item	Calories	Protein (grams)	Carb. (grams)	Fat (grams)	Chol. (mg)	Fiber (grams)	Sodium (mg)
Tempeh	395	38*	34	15	0	6	12
Tofu	150	16*	4	9	0	1	14
Beef	798	43	0	68	179	0	127
Chicken	386	58	0	15	166	0	138
Tuna (low-sodium)	271	53	0	5	83	0	250

*Soy protein

SOY-BASED FOODS

The following soy-based foods are useful—or, in the case of soy sauce—essential in a well-stocked pantry, but don't count on them to supply protein or genistein. They do have an important advantage over their non-soy counterparts, which is that none of them contains any saturated fat or cholesterol.

Egg replacers: Made from potato starch and lecithin, a soy product, egg replacers have the same emulsifying properties as eggs. Egg replacers do not supply genistein or other nutrients, but unlike eggs, they contain no cholesterol. This powder is usually available only in health food stores and should not be confused with liquid, egg-based egg substitutes sold in the dairy case in supermarkets. Mixed with water, egg replacers can be used in place of eggs in baked goods. Unrefrigerated, the powder keeps for six months.

Soy margarine: This is margarine made primarily or entirely from soy oil. Its advantage over other types of margarine or butter is that it contains no saturated fat. It does not, however, provide genistein or soy protein. Many commercial margarines are made primarily of soy oil and are widely available in supermarkets. Use sparingly, as you would any fat. They generally last about three months under refrigeration.

Soy mayonnaise: All commercial mayonnaises are made with soybean oil. Most contain eggs, although you can find eggless varieties. There is also a commercial tofu-based mayonnaise, made by Nasoya brands, that has no saturated fat or eggs. Tofu-based mayonnaise, either homemade or commercial, is a healthier choice than oil-based mayonnaise because it is lower in fat. However, it provides only a trace of soy protein or genistein. Ordinary and low-fat mayonnaises are, of course, found in supermarkets; look for Nasoya in health-food markets. I include a simple recipe for homemade Tofu Mayonnaise (page 59).

Use tofu-based mayonnaise just as you would the regular type—in salads and on sandwiches. All mayonnaise and foods made with mayonnaise should be refrigerated. Commercial mayonnaise will last up to three months in the refrigerator; homemade tofu mayonnaise kept in a sealed container should be consumed within a month and foods made with mayonnaise should be consumed within a week.

Soybean oil: Soybean oil is extracted from whole soybeans (the leftover protein solids go into animal feed) and sold as pure soybean oil, or as an ingredient in vegetable oil, or processed into margarines and shortenings. Like soy margarine, soybean oil has no saturated fat, but it does not provide soy protein or genistein. Soybean oil is sold in the cooking oil section of supermarkets and health food stores. Many familiar brands, such as Wesson, are 100 percent soybean oil.

Use soy oil for sautéing or frying and any other way in which you would use cooking oil. It can be used in salad dressings, if desired, although olive oil has more flavor. Stored in the pantry, it should be used within six months once opened.

Soy sauce: Soy sauce is a condiment made from fermented soybeans and wheat flour. Tamari, shoyu, and teriyaki sauces are very similar to soy sauce, but none of these condiments contains genistein or soy protein. These condiments may be found in grocery stores and are easy to add to Chinese and Japanese foods. They are also delicious in marinades and Asian-style salad dressings. These sauces are all very high in sodium (even the reduced-salt varieties) and should be used sparingly.

There is a tremendous amount
of discussion these days over
the merits of vegetable protein
relative to animal protein. The
basic difference is that animal
protein is complete all by
itself, while vegetable proteins
need to be combined with
other foods to create complete
proteins. In other words, animal protein provides all the
essential amino acids for tissue growth and repair, while
the protein found in soybeans
does not contain all the essential amino acids. Animal protein, however, contains high
levels of saturated fat and cholesterol, which in the opinion of
many doctors and nutritionists
far outweighs its benefits.
Since it is very easy to com-
pensate for the incomplete
protein from vegetable
sources, it is clear that, from a
health standpoint, vegetable
protein is the superior choice.

How do you obtain complete
protein from vegetable
sources? Cultures around the
world, from primitive to
advanced, have known the
answer to that question for
ages. Mexicans eat pinto beans
with corn tortillas; Indians eat
lentils with rice; Native
Americans ate corn and beans;
Chinese consume bean curd
with rice. When beans are consumed together with grains,
these two foods provide all the
amino acids necessary to form
a complete protein.

how to get optimum nutrition from soy

If you are concerned about following today's accepted standards for a healthy diet, you try to eat foods with high levels of complex carbohydrates and moderate to low amounts of fat. You obtain nearly all your protein from plant sources. Soy fulfills all those guidelines, and more. Providing the highest levels of protein available from plant sources, it is cholesterol free and full of vitamins, minerals, and fiber.

You can see for yourself how soy foods fit into your healthy lifestyle by using the nutritional analysis included at the end of each of my recipes. You'll be able to determine just how many grams of soy protein a given dish provides, its calorie count, and the amount of carbohydrate, fat, cholesterol, fiber, and sodium it contains. Let's look more closely at what this means, especially as it relates to soy.

CALORIES

Most soy products pack a big nutritional wallop for the number of calories they contain. In nutritional lingo, they are considered high nutrient-density foods, in contrast to, say, a candy bar, which contains low levels of nutrients but has a high calorie count.

Calories are a measurement of the amount of energy a food yields. The only nutrients that provide calories are proteins, carbohydrates, and fats. Vitamins, minerals, and water have no calories but are essential to the body in other ways. Calories are measured by the heat that is released when the food is metabolized. Your metabolism, or the rate at which you metabolize food, is related to height, age, weight, and hereditary factors. You need to consume a sufficient number of high-quality calories to give you energy for your body's daily needs, but not so much that your body stores the excess as fat. Soy is one of nature's most efficient foods because it provides a high level of nutrition at a relatively low caloric cost.

PROTEIN

Found in both animal and plant sources, protein contains the essential building blocks that allow our bodies to grow and injuries to heal. Humans cannot survive without it. Soy foods, which provide the highest levels of protein available from plant sources, are unique because they provide the miraculous nutrient genistein in addition to other nutrients needed for growth and tissue repair. Remember, to receive the disease-preventing benefits of genistein, doctors recommend consuming at least 25 grams of soy protein a day. Protein contains 4 calories per gram.

CARBOHYDRATES

There are both simple and complex carbohydrates. Candy, fruit, refined flours, and all sugars are simple carbohydrates. Whole grains, vegetables, and legumes—and of course that includes soybeans—are complex carbohydrates. These days, doctors and nutritionists advise that the bulk of a healthy diet should come from this latter group.

Carbohydrates provide energy by breaking down into glucose (simple sugar) in the bloodstream. Insulin is released by the pancreas as needed to absorb glucose in the body. If there is a slight excess of glucose in the bloodstream, it will be stored in the muscles as potential energy. If there is a tremendous excess of glucose in the bloodstream that isn't used readily for the body's energy needs, it is converted into fat. Complex carbohydrates provide many nutrients, and unlike candy and sweets, they are not likely to create excessive glucose in the bloodstream. Soy foods are ideal complex carbohydrates because they have a high nutrient density and their consumption results in low levels of blood sugar. Carbohydrates yield 4 calories per gram.

FAT

Today's nutritional guidelines suggest eating a diet low in fat. That fat should be mostly, if not entirely, obtained from plant sources. A diet dependent on soy foods will naturally include no more than a healthy allowance of fat. Fat is a necessary nutrient. It protects the lining of every cell in our body;

I have provided serving suggestions with the recipes in this book to help you obtain sufficient high-quality protein. For example, I would recommend that you have Black Bean Chili with Tempeh (page 135) with a piece of Soy Cheese Corn Bread (page 99). Or Tofu Cacciatore (page 142) with Spanish Brown Rice Pilaf (page 182). Or the sauce for Penne with Soy Sausage Bolognese (page 176) over Soy Polenta (page 184); or Soy Cheese Pizza (page 110), with its delicious whole wheat crust supporting a gooey soy cheese topping. As you'll see, properly combining grains and beans is a snap.

it emulsifies food for digestion; it provides a layer of protection for the body against harsh temperatures and physical harm; its concentrated energy may save us in times of starvation. Fat only becomes "bad" when it is consumed in larger quantities than we need, since fats are higher in calories than protein and carbohydrates.

Animal fats are saturated (solid at room temperature) and contain cholesterol. Saturated fats and cholesterol are the culprits in heart disease, cancer, high blood pressure, and strokes because they can build up in the bloodstream and block the flow of blood to the heart. With rare exceptions, such as palm oil and coconut oil, fats from plants are unsaturated and cholesterol free: a much healthier choice in the diet. A diet high in soy will automatically be low in saturated fat. Fat is measured in grams and yields 9 calories per gram.

CHOLESTEROL

Soy foods are free of cholesterol, a substance which in excess may contribute to heart disease. Cholesterol is primarly found in animal products; with rare exceptions, plants do not contain it. A good nutritional guideline is to limit intake of cholesterol to no more than 400 milligrams per day.

FIBER

Eating complex carbohydrates, such as soybeans, will automatically give you the fiber that you need to maintain good health. Dietary fiber is the nondigestible part of a carbohydrate, usually derived from the bran, stems, leaves, seeds, or peels of fruits, vegetables, and grains. Fiber aids in food digestion; it cannot be broken down by the human body and so it cleans out residue in the digestive tract as it works its way through the body. A diet high in fiber can help prevent diseases of the digestive tract, from diverticulitis to colon cancer. Nutritionists recommend consuming 15 grams of fiber each day.

SODIUM

The body requires only very small amounts of sodium, which it uses to keep the bloodstream functioning properly. It is very difficult, however, to keep the level of sodium in your diet low because sodium occurs naturally in many foods. Furthermore, when food is processed, sodium is added to almost everything. When there is too much sodium in the bloodstream, the body reacts by increasing the blood pressure. Prolonged periods of elevated blood pressure can result in cardiovascular diseases, such as strokes, heart attacks, and aneurysms.

Most soy foods are naturally low in sodium; in fact, the sodium content in animal products is in general much higher than in plant-based foods, such as soy. The sodium content of processed foods is also much higher than that of fresh foods. Drinking a sufficient quantity of water daily (eight glasses) may help reduce sodium in the bloodstream. Sodium consumption should not exceed 3,000 milligrams (3 grams) per day.

n u t r i t i o n   i n f o r m a t i o n

Now that you understand how nutritional terms apply to soy foods, let's look at a recipe analysis. I've chosen a hearty main course, Black Bean Chili with Tempeh (page 135), as an example. The chart below provides all the essential information you will need for healthy meal planning.

First, look for the quantity of soy protein. You'll see that this recipe contains 6 grams of soy protein out of a total of 13 grams of protein. That 6 grams can be calculated as part of your daily 25 grams of soy protein.

Black Bean Chili with Tempeh

Nutritional values are per serving. Serving size is approximately 6 ounces.

Calories	Total Protein	Soy Protein	Carbohydrate	Fat	Cholesterol	Fiber	Sodium
207	13 g	6 g	30 g	4.5 g	0 mg	7 g	9 mg

Notice that this recipe contains zero cholesterol and plenty of fiber. It is low in fat and sodium. The calorie count for this filling, healthful meal is also surprisingly low.

A chart just like this one follows each of my full recipes, so you can easily see exactly how much beneficial soy protein you are consuming as you pick and choose your favorite foods.

These nutritional analyses make it simple to ensure that you consume 25 grams of soy protein a day. And as you will see, it is not hard to do at all, since 25 grams adds up very quickly. How quickly? For starters, try these simple suggestions. You won't notice a difference in your daily diet, and you'll get an instant, painless head start on your daily "dose" of soy protein.

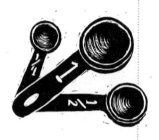

Have your breakfast cereal with soy milk (6.6 grams of soy protein per cup).

Snack on soy cheese with crackers (6 grams of soy protein per ounce).

Add a fruity soy yogurt to your lunch (12 grams of soy protein per cup).

Dress your salad with a soy-based dressing (2 to 5 grams of soy protein per serving).

Sprinkle soy parmesan on your pasta (2 grams of soy protein per 2 teaspoons).

- Treat yourself to a commercial, frozen soy-based dessert (around 8 grams of soy protein per serving, depending on the product).

A little planning will help ensure you get all the health benefits associated with soy and genistein. The following section offers a week's worth of sample menus, all designed to give you the 25 essential grams of soy protein each day. You have *plenty* of free choice—most meals in this sample week's menu are completely up to you (although you could certainly fill those free slots with some soy foods, too!).

Sunday—26 grams of soy protein

BREAKFAST: Tofu Florentine (page 89) with a Cream Scone (page 87) (15 grams)

LUNCH: Soy Caesar Salad (page 53) (2) and entree of your choice

DINNER: Appetizer and entree of your choice; Soy Tiramisù (page 204) for dessert (9)

Monday—31 grams of soy protein

BREAKFAST: Fruit, cereal, or other items of your choice

LUNCH: Spinach Salad with Warm Soy Bacon Dressing (page 52) (10) and Black Bean Chili with Tempeh (page 135) (6) with Soy Cheese Corn Bread (page 99) (3)

DINNER: Salad, Roasted Vegetable and Soy Cheese Napoleons (page 44) (12), dessert of your choice

Tuesday—26 grams of soy protein

BREAKFAST: Fruit, cereal, or other items of your choice

LUNCH: Tempeh Picnic Salad (page 66) (26)

DINNER: Appetizer, entree, and dessert of your choice

Wednesday—31 grams of soy protein

BREAKFAST: Soy Nut Granola with Soy Milk (page 84) (15)

LUNCH: Entree of your choice and 2 ounces of soy cheese (10)

DINNER: Tofu Basil Soup (page 120) (6) and entree of your choice

Thursday—38 grams of soy protein

BREAKFAST: Fruit, cereal, or other items of your choice

LUNCH: Soy Tortellini Salad (page 71) (10) and Carrot Ginger Soy Soup (page 123) (4)

DINNER: Salad, Tempeh Fajitas (page 152) (21), Tofu Flan (page 205) (11)

Friday—28 grams of soy protein

BREAKFAST: Curried Tofu with Red Peppers and Onions (page 86) (19) and Soy Milk Pancakes (page 85) (2)

LUNCH: Broccoli Tempeh Salad (page 70) (7)

DINNER: Appetizer, entree, and dessert of your choice

Saturday—27 grams of soy protein

BREAKFAST: Tofu, Spinach, and Soy Ham Quiche (page 88) (11)

LUNCH: Appetizer and entree of your choice

DINNER: Salad, Penne with Soy Sausage Bolognese (page 176) (16) and dessert of your choice

This fun and flexible week's worth of meal ideas proves that you won't have to make radical changes in your eating habits to reap the benefits of soy. Whether you're a vegan, lacto-vegetarian, lacto-ovo-vegetarian, semi-vegetarian, or just interested in adding soy products to a conventional healthy diet, I guarantee you'll be delighted by how deliciously soy fits into your life.

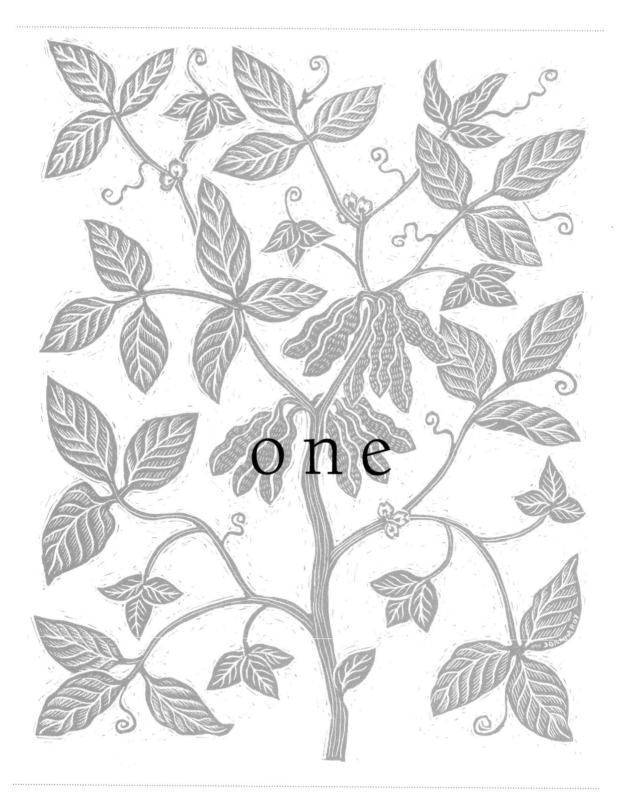

one

appetizers, dips, and spreads

Can you entertain—or simply snack—and still make sure you get your 25 grams of soy protein? Of course! Soy products—from cheeses to soy "ham" and "sausage" to tofu and tempeh—make fabulous appetizers. Low in fat, free of cholesterol, and crammed with the goodness of soy, they are easy to use and flexible in taste.

The appetizers in this chapter range from the simple to the exotic. Try the effortless Soy Caprese—sliced soy mozzarella with ripe tomatoes, basil, and a drizzle of fragrant olive oil. Or the rewarding Soy Gyoza-Tempeh Pot Stickers. Serve these tasty sesame-scented Asian dumplings as a first course or as part of a buffet with Tempeh Spring Rolls with Sweet-and-Sour Sauce and Crispy Tofu with Plum and Ginger Sauce. You can make a whole meal of yummy appetizers: vegetable crudités with Scandinavian Dill Dip; warm-from-the-oven Soy Sausage Rolls; and aromatic Marinated Eggplant Stuffed with Soy Cream Cheese.

You can make a party favorite, like Tofu Guacamole, that's as rich and creamy as the original. Or feel free to experiment: that's how I came up with the incredible Roasted Vegetable and Soy Cheese Napoleons. I saw something like them at a dinner, and I couldn't wait to get home and whip up a soy version of these layers of puffy pastry, oven-browned vegetables, and warm melted soy mozzarella.

Soy appetizers make simple snacks, casual dinners, or lavish buffets as nutritious as they are delicious. Your guests or family won't even know they're getting healthful food.

Soy Caprese

Nothing is more natural than the flavor combination of ripe red tomatoes with pungent fresh basil. With the addition of protein-packed soy mozzarella and crunchy cucumbers, this take-off on a classic Italian appetizer is a wholesome start to any meal and is pretty enough to serve when entertaining. Simply slice all the ingredients thin and even, arrange on a plate in a circle, and drizzle with a little of your best olive oil.

1 medium cucumber, thinly sliced

8 ounces soy mozzarella, thinly sliced

3 roma tomatoes, thinly sliced

6 basil leaves, shredded

Extra-virgin olive oil, as needed

1. On a serving platter, arrange the cucumber, cheese slices, and tomato slices in concentric circles, overlapping them like shingles. Sprinkle with the shredded basil and chill.

2. Drizzle a little olive oil on top before serving.

SERVES 6 AS AN APPETIZER

Calories	Total Protein	Soy Protein	Carbohydrate	Fat	Cholesterol	Fiber	Sodium
100	6 g	6 g	4.5 g	7 g	0 mg	2 g	195 mg

Information is per serving.

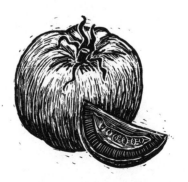

Crispy Tofu with Plum and Ginger Sauce

Smooth tofu gets a crisp, brown crust in this Japanese-inspired delicacy. The warm tofu is then swathed in a flavorful plum-ginger sauce for a dish with both memorable taste and texture. You can cut the tofu into large slices for an appetizer or light meal or into small bite-size chunks for hors d'oeuvres.

Plum and Ginger Sauce

4 cups Vegetable Stock (page 120)

½ cup plum jam

1 tablespoon soy sauce

1 1-inch piece fresh ginger, peeled and minced

2 tablespoons apricot preserves

2 pounds firm tofu

½ cup whole wheat flour

4 tablespoons cornstarch

½ cup vegetable oil

¼ cup sesame seeds

1. Bring the stock to a boil and add the plum jam, soy sauce, and ginger. Stir vigorously to dissolve the jam.

2. Let the stock boil once again and add the apricot preserves. Lower heat and simmer, uncovered, until the mixture is reduced to a slightly syrupy consistency, about 30 minutes. (Makes 3 cups; reserve 1½ cups for tofu. Extra sauce keeps, refrigerated, for about 1 month.)

3. Meanwhile, slice each pound of tofu into 16 slices (or into bite-size cubes for hors d'oeuvres). In a large bowl, combine the flour and cornstarch and coat the tofu slices evenly with the mixture.

4. Heat the oil in a large frying pan and add only as many pieces of tofu as will fit without crowding. Brown them evenly and set aside on absorbent paper. Continue until all the tofu is cooked.

5. Place 4 pieces on each plate and pour about 3 tablespoons of plum sauce over each serving. Sprinkle with sesame seeds and serve at once.

SERVES 8 AS A FIRST COURSE OR
MAKES 32 HORS D'OEUVRES

Calories	Total Protein	Soy Protein	Carbohydrate	Fat	Cholesterol	Fiber	Sodium
236	11.3 g	9 g	29.1 g	10 g	0 mg	3.1 g	140 mg

Information is per entree serving. *Note:* For hors d'oeuvres, the dipping sauce can go into an extra bowl on the side.

Soy Gyoza-Tempeh Pot Stickers

Pot stickers are traditional Chinese dumplings, stuffed and then sautéed or steamed. They usually contain pork or shrimp, but you won't miss the meat with this delicious soy filling that features both tempeh and tofu in a sesame-and-garlic–flavored sauce. Serve with other Asian-inspired dishes, such as Crispy Tofu with Plum and Ginger Sauce (page 35) or Szechuan Tempeh (page 150), or with a salad as a light meal.

½ pound tempeh, finely diced

12 ounces extra-firm tofu, crumbled

1 cup shredded green cabbage

2 scallions, white and tender green parts, chopped

1 garlic clove, finely minced

1 ½-inch piece fresh ginger, peeled and finely minced

2 tablespoons toasted sesame oil

2 tablespoons soy sauce

30 pot sticker wrappers (available in deli cases of large grocery stores, health food stores, or Asian markets)

2 tablespoons vegetable oil

Plum and Ginger Sauce (optional, see recipe, page 35)

Sesame seeds to garnish

1. In a medium bowl, combine the tempeh, tofu, cabbage, scallions, garlic, and ginger.

2. In a skillet, heat the sesame oil over medium-high heat and add the tempeh mixture. Sauté until scallions are soft, about 5 minutes. Add the soy sauce and cook for 2 more minutes.

3. Place 1 teaspoon of the cooked mixture in the center of a pot sticker wrapper. Moisten the edges with water and fold the wrapper in half over the filling. Press the edges with your fingers to seal the dough.

4. Heat the vegetable oil over medium heat in a large skillet. (You can use 2 skillets simultaneously to speed the process.) Add as many pot stickers as will fit without crowding and cook over medium heat approximately 2 minutes or until browned on the bottom.

5. Add about ⅓ cup of water to the pan or pans; cover, and cook for 4 to 5 minutes or until the liquid has cooked away. Place the pot stickers, browned side up, on a warm serving platter and sprinkle with sesame seeds. Serve with sauce, if desired.

SERVES 6

Calories	Total Protein	Soy Protein	Carbohydrate	Fat	Cholesterol	Fiber	Sodium
150	8 g	5 g	7.5 g	10 g	2.5 mg	1 g	289 mg

Information is for 5 pot stickers.

Tofu Guacamole

As your family and friends sample this rich, creamy guacamole, they'll never know they're getting soy protein as well. Pureed tofu blends seamlessly into this avocado dip: everyone's favorite complement to chips or raw vegetables. It also makes a wonderful topping for South of the Border Tofu Salad (page 61).

> 1 ripe, medium avocado
> 8 ounces extra-firm tofu
> 4 tablespoons chunky salsa

1. Peel, seed, and mash the avocado.
2. Put the avocado and tofu in a food processor or blender and mix until thoroughly combined.
3. Scrape into a serving bowl and fold in the salsa. Serve at room temperature. Do not make guacamole more than 1 hour in advance, as it will turn brown.

MAKES ABOUT 2 CUPS; 16 1-OUNCE (2 TABLESPOONS) SERVINGS

Calories	Total Protein	Soy Protein	Carbohydrate	Fat	Cholesterol	Fiber	Sodium
65	3.7 g	3.7 g	3 g	5 g	0 mg	1.6 g	43 mg

Information is for a 1-ounce serving.

Easy Entertaining

Having a few friends over? Did a few unexpected guests drop by? No problem—with a few basic soy products on hand, you can whip up these quick, delicious appetizers and snacks in no time. In addition to making good eating, these tidbits make good sense. One almond cream cheese ball, for example, provides 2.6 grams of soy protein.

almond soy cream cheese balls

Toast ½ cup of slivered almonds over high heat and chop them fine. Scoop 8 ounces of chilled soy cream cheese into small balls using a teaspoon or melon baller. Roll balls in the toasted almonds. Chill and serve.

soy cream cheese with papaya pear chutney

Soften 8 ounces of soy cream cheese and beat into it 1 cup of Papaya Pear Chutney (page 140) for a creamy, tangy spread to serve with crackers. Or, line a plate with lettuce leaves, put the cream cheese on top, and smother it with the chutney. Surround this with crackers or small bread toasts.

Tempeh Spring Rolls with Sweet-and-Sour Sauce

Everybody loves traditional Chinese spring rolls. In this version, tempeh replaces the usual shrimp or pork, making a light, crispy spring roll that's every bit as satisfying as the original, even as it provides 8 grams of soy protein. The accompanying sauce rounds out the flavors. These spring rolls are wonderful as snacks or appetizers on their own, or they go well with other Asian-inspired dishes such as the Soy Gyoza-Tempeh Pot Stickers (page 36) and Kung Pao Tempeh (page 148).

8 ounces tempeh

2 tablespoons toasted sesame oil

2 tablespoons soy sauce

3 scallions, white and tender green parts, sliced

2 garlic cloves, minced

1 1-inch piece fresh ginger, grated

¼ head green cabbage, shredded

4 large carrots, shredded

4 fresh mushrooms, thinly sliced

1 cup Vegetable Stock (page 120)

½ teaspoon salt

½ teaspoon black pepper

8 wonton wrappers, at room temperature (available in deli cases of large grocery stores, health food stores, or Asian markets)

¼ cup soy milk

1 cup vegetable oil, or as needed

1 recipe Sweet and Sour Sauce (page 39)

1. With the tempeh at room temperature, crumble it into small pieces.

2. In a large skillet or wok, heat the sesame oil and soy sauce over high heat and sauté the scallions, garlic, and ginger for 15 seconds.

3. Lower the temperature slightly and add the cabbage, carrots, mushrooms, and tempeh. Sauté for 3 more minutes, adding stock as needed to prevent sticking, and remove from the heat. Season with salt and pepper.

4. Fill each wrapper with 3 even tablespoons of filling, and fold up from the bottom and both sides. Roll over to enclose the filling, and brush with soy milk to seal.

5. Fill a deep-fryer or wok with vegetable oil to a depth of 1½ inches. Heat to 375°F., measured on a deep-fat thermometer, and fry each spring roll for 1 minute on each side or until golden brown. Remove from oil and place on paper towels to absorb excess oil. Serve hot. Garnish with Sweet and Sour Sauce.

SERVES 8

Calories	Total Protein	Soy Protein	Carbohydrate	Fat	Cholesterol	Fiber	Sodium
330	8 g	8 g	15 g	27 g	0 mg	3.4 g	409 mg

Information is for 1 spring roll.

Sweet and Sour Sauce

2 tablespoons vegetable oil

1 medium onion, chopped

3 celery stalks, chopped

2 medium red bell peppers, chopped

2 garlic cloves, minced

½ cup white wine vinegar

½ cup brown sugar, loosely packed

1 cup ketchup

1 cup canned crushed pineapple

¼ cup pineapple juice, as needed

1. Heat the oil in a large saucepan over medium-high heat. Add the onion, celery, and peppers and sauté until the onion is translucent, about 5 minutes. Lower the heat, add the garlic, and sauté for 1 more minute.

2. Add the vinegar, brown sugar, ketchup, and crushed pineapple, stirring well after each addition.

3. Simmer the mixture for 30 minutes, adding pineapple juice as needed if sauce becomes too thick. (Extra sauce keeps in the refrigerator, tightly sealed, for up to 2 weeks.)

MAKES ABOUT 4 CUPS

Calories	Total Protein	Soy Protein	Carbohydrate	Fat	Cholesterol	Fiber	Sodium
125	1 g	0 g	24 g	3.5 g	0 mg	1 g	198 mg

Information is for 1 ounce.

crudités with assorted dips

On a flat basket or tray, place 2 or 3 small bowls of assorted dips, such as Spicy Tofu Peanut Sauce (see recipe, page 178), Creamy Garlic Dressing (see recipe, page 54), or Scandinavian Dill Dip (page 43). Surround the bowls with decoratively arranged carrot and celery sticks, broccoli florets, red and yellow pepper strips, jicama sticks, sugar snap peas, and radishes.

santa fe nachos

For a quick and hearty appetizer, spread a bag of corn chips on a cookie sheet. Spoon over them 3 cups of Soybean Chili (page 134) or Black Bean Chili with Tempeh (page 135). Cover with 8 ounces of shredded soy cheddar cheese and bake for 5 to 7 minutes. Remove to a platter and serve, along with salsa.

Browning with Soy Milk

Nothing is more appetizing than golden-brown pastries or rolls fresh from the oven. But how to get that golden glow? The traditional method is to brush the tops of baked goods with raw egg, beaten lightly with a little water, but I have discovered that soy milk works just as well. Using a pastry brush, lightly paint the tops of pastries or breads with a wash of soy milk before baking. The crusts brown beautifully—and there's no added cholesterol.

Soy Sausage Rolls

This recipe makes crunchy, bite-size spirals of tasty soy sausage wrapped in a golden crust. Served warm from the oven, they are impossible to resist. The recipe can be easily doubled, if desired, and prepared ahead. Bake the rolls just before serving so they will be at their crisp best.

> 1 10-inch sheet pre-made puff pastry
> ¼ cup soy milk
> 1 14-ounce package ground soy sausage
> ½ small onion, chopped

1. Thaw the pastry for 30 minutes. Preheat the oven to 400°F.
2. Unfold the pastry onto a flat surface and brush it with the soy milk.
3. Crumble the sausage and spread it evenly over the entire surface of the pastry. Strew the chopped onion on top.
4. Roll the pastry up, jelly-roll style, and cut crosswise into 18 slices. Place on a baking sheet lined with parchment paper and brush the tops with the remaining soy milk.
5. Bake for 15 minutes or until pastry is slightly browned.

MAKES 18

Calories	Total Protein	Soy Protein	Carbohydrate	Fat	Cholesterol	Fiber	Sodium
128	6.5 g	3.5 g	9.1 g	4.8 g	0 mg	1.6 g	1435 mg

Information is for 1 sausage roll.

Spinach Cheese Rolls

These crispy, bite-size spirals of spinach and cheese in a golden crust are great for a large group because the recipe can be doubled easily and prepared in advance. They must be baked just before serving, however, to be at their airy, golden best.

    1 10-inch sheet pre-made puff pastry

    1 10-ounce package frozen chopped spinach

    6 ounces soy mozzarella cheese, grated

    ¼ cup soy parmesan cheese

    1 small leek, minced, white only

    1 garlic clove, minced

    ¼ cup soy milk, or as needed

1. Thaw the pastry for 30 minutes. Preheat the oven to 400°F.

2. Thaw the spinach. Squeeze by handfuls to remove excess water. Combine the spinach, cheeses, leek, and garlic in a bowl and set aside.

3. Unfold the pastry onto a flat surface and brush with soy milk.

4. Top the entire surface with the spinach mixture and, beginning on a long side, roll up jelly-roll style. Cut crosswise into 18 slices. Brush with soy milk and place on a parchment-lined cookie sheet.

5. Bake for 15 minutes or until golden brown.

MAKES 18

Calories	Total Protein	Soy Protein	Carbohydrate	Fat	Cholesterol	Fiber	Sodium
97	5 g	4.7 g	6 g	5.3 g	0 mg	1 g	120 mg

Information is for 1 spinach roll.

Marinated Eggplant Stuffed with Soy Cream Cheese

Inspired by a traditional Provençal dish, this delicious appetizer is easy to assemble. Sautéed eggplant slices are rolled around a soy cheese filling and then marinated in an herb-infused vinaigrette. Serve whole or sliced. They keep in the refrigerator for up to three days, gaining in flavor as they marinate.

2 medium eggplants

2 teaspoons salt

1 cup olive oil

8 ounces soy cream cheese

⅓ cup red wine vinegar

3 garlic cloves, minced

¼ cup chopped Italian parsley

2 sprigs of oregano

⅓ cup chopped fresh basil

⅛ teaspoon salt

⅛ teaspoon pepper

1. Trim the stems and ends from the eggplants and cut each into ⅛-inch-thick slices. There should be about 24 slices. Line several cookie sheets with paper towels and lay the slices on them. Sprinkle the slices with salt and let them drain for 30 minutes. Rinse the eggplant and pat dry.

2. In a large sauté pan, heat 2 tablespoons of olive oil and sauté 6 eggplant slices at a time until they are golden brown, 2 to 3 minutes per side. Set the cooked slices aside on paper towels. Adding 2 tablespoons of oil for each batch, continue until all the eggplant has been browned.

3. Spread each slice of eggplant with 1 tablespoon of the cheese and roll up the eggplant slice. Tightly pack them, skewered with a toothpick, seam side down so they don't unroll, in a shallow baking pan.

4. In a small bowl, whisk together the remaining olive oil, vinegar, garlic, parsley, oregano, basil, and salt and pepper. Pour over the eggplant rolls to marinate.

5. Place in refrigerator and marinate overnight, up to 3 days. Serve chilled or at room temperature.

SERVES 6 (3 TO 4 PIECES PER PERSON) AS AN APPETIZER OR MAKES 24 HORS D'OEUVRES

Calories	Total Protein	Soy Protein	Carbohydrate	Fat	Cholesterol	Fiber	Sodium
115	1 g	1 g	3 g	11 g	0 mg	1 g	46 mg

Information is for 1 piece.

Scandinavian Dill Dip

Inspired by Swedish smorgasbords, where fresh dill infuses sauces for salmon, herring, meats, and vegetables, this tangy dip brings out the best in raw vegetables. It's great drizzled over steamed or roasted vegetables or a mixed green salad.

> 1 cup plain soy yogurt
>
> 2 tablespoons red wine vinegar
>
> 1 teaspoon chopped fresh dill
>
> 2 teaspoons sugar
>
> White pepper to taste

1. Combine all the ingredients in a small bowl and mix well.
2. Cover and chill until serving.

MAKES ABOUT 1 CUP; 8 1-OUNCE (2 TABLESPOONS) SERVINGS

Calories	Total Protein	Soy Protein	Carbohydrate	Fat	Cholesterol	Fiber	Sodium
29	1 g	1 g	11 g	0 g	0 mg	1 g	2.5 mg

Information is for a 1-ounce serving.

Roasted Vegetable and
Soy Cheese Napoleons

Inspired by Napoleons—those rich, layered French pastries—I've created this beautiful but deceptively easy to prepare dish. It features flavorful roasted vegetables and thin slices of soy mozzarella alternated with golden circles of pre-made puff pastry. Serve warm from the oven, so the cheese bubbles and runs.

4 10-inch sheets pre-made puff
  pastry, defrosted
1 large eggplant
1 teaspoon salt
1 large zucchini
1 large yellow squash
1 ripe, large tomato

¼ cup olive oil
Italian seasoning to taste
12 ounces soy mozzarella cheese,
  cut into 12 slices
6 sprigs of rosemary, about 3 to
  5 inches long, to be used as
  skewers

1. Preheat the oven to 400°F. Line a large baking sheet with parchment paper.

2. With a 3½-inch round cookie cutter, cut the pastry dough into 12 circles and place on the baking sheet. Pierce each circle all over with the tines of a fork and bake for 15 minutes. Remove from oven and set aside.

3. Trim the stem and end of the eggplant and slice crosswise into 12 slices. Lay the slices on paper towels and sprinkle with salt. Let them exude their juices for about 30 minutes and pat them dry.

4. Slice the zucchini and yellow squash lengthwise into 6 slices each.

5. Slice the tomato. Arrange it and the eggplant, zucchini, and squash slices in one layer on baking sheets. Brush them with olive oil and sprinkle Italian seasoning on top.

6. Roast for 12 to 15 minutes, until vegetables are browned. Remove from oven to cool. (The vegetables can be roasted a day ahead and refrigerated, tightly wrapped, until ready to use.)

7. Place a round of puff pastry on a baking sheet and on top of it layer the Napoleon in the following order: eggplant, zucchini, soy mozzarella, tomato, yellow squash, eggplant, soy mozzarella, puff pastry. Skewer the Napoleon from top to bottom with a wooden pick to hold it together. Repeat for the remaining 5 Napoleons.

8. With the oven still at 400°F., bake the Napoleons for 5 minutes, or until the cheese is melted. Remove the wooden pick, replacing it with a rosemary sprig, and serve immediately.

SERVES 6

Calories	Total Protein	Soy Protein	Carbohydrate	Fat	Cholesterol	Fiber	Sodium
317	14 g	12 g	15 g	22 g	0 mg	2 g	933 mg

Information is for 1 Napoleon.

Soy Almond Butter

This nutty spread makes a great filling for sandwiches or dip for bread, crackers, vegetables, and fruit. I have even used it as a filling in a layer cake. Use low-fat soy milk in this recipe because the almonds are high in fat.

> 2 cups whole almonds
> ½ cup low-fat soy milk
> ⅛ teaspoon salt

1. Place the almonds in one layer on a baking sheet and toast in a 350°F. oven for about 8 minutes, watching carefully as they will burn easily. Let cool slightly.
2. In a food processor or blender, grind the almonds to a fine powder. With the processor running, gradually add the soy milk and salt until the mixture reaches a smooth, spreadable consistency. The spread keeps for 2 days refrigerated in an airtight container.

MAKES 1½ CUPS; 12 1-OUNCE (2 TABLESPOONS) SERVINGS

Calories	Total Protein	Soy Protein	Carbohydrate	Fat	Cholesterol	Fiber	Sodium
131	4.5 g	0.5 g	4.5 g	11.5 g	0 mg	2.6 g	25 mg

Information is for a 1-ounce serving.

Cucumber Raita

This is a soy version of one of India's best known side dishes, a refreshing blend of yogurt and diced cucumber seasoned with mint and cumin. It's often served with flat bread for dipping to accompany hot and spicy main courses. Try it with Tofu Curry (page 140). It makes a great vegetable dip, too.

1 cup plain soy yogurt
1 medium cucumber
2 mint leaves, chopped
½ teaspoon ground cumin
½ teaspoon salt
White pepper to taste

1. Peel the cucumber and cut in half lengthwise. Scoop out the seeds with a spoon.
2. Finely dice the cucumber, place in a colander, and let excess juice drain for a few minutes.
3. Combine the cucumber, yogurt, mint leaves, and cumin in a medium bowl. Mix thoroughly and season with salt and pepper.

MAKES ABOUT 1½ CUPS; 12 1-OUNCE (2 TABLESPOONS) SERVINGS

Calories	Total Protein	Soy Protein	Carbohydrate	Fat	Cholesterol	Fiber	Sodium
30	1 g	1 g	11 g	0 g	0 mg	1.5 g	16 mg

Information is for a 1-ounce serving.

Cheddar Nut Spread

Macadamia nuts give this spread a luxurious richness. Pecans work just as well. Try this on crackers or pita bread, or with celery sticks or endive leaves for a delicious appetizer or snack.

2½ cups soy cream cheese

¼ cup chopped macadamia nuts

¼ cup shredded soy cheddar cheese (about 2 ounces)

1. Bring the cream cheese to room temperature. With an electric beater at high speed, whip it until fluffy, about 5 minutes.

2. Mix the cream cheese with the nuts and soy cheddar until thoroughly combined. Chill.

MAKES ABOUT 3 CUPS; 24 1-OUNCE (2 TABLESPOONS) SERVINGS

Calories	Total Protein	Soy Protein	Carbohydrate	Fat	Cholesterol	Fiber	Sodium
100	2 g	1.5 g	1 g	9.5 g	0 mg	2.6 g	142 mg

Information is for a 1-ounce serving.

Strawberry Soy Spread

This spread does wonders for a slice of toasted Soy Whole Wheat Bread (page 106) or warm Soy Milk Biscuits (page 94).

2 cups soy cream cheese

½ cup soy margarine

¼ cup strawberry jam

1. Soften the soy cream cheese and margarine to room temperature. With an electric beater at high speed, whip the cream cheese and margarine until it is fluffy, about 5 minutes.

2. Mix in the jam until thoroughly combined. Chill.

MAKES 3 CUPS; 24 1-OUNCE (1 GENEROUS TABLESPOON) SERVINGS

Calories	Total Protein	Soy Protein	Carbohydrate	Fat	Cholesterol	Fiber	Sodium
117	2 g	1 g	2 g	11 g	0 mg	0 g	139 mg

Information is for a 1-ounce serving.

Homemade Soy Nut Butters

Love the taste of peanut butter? Got a food processor? It's so easy to make your own nut butter: just combine four parts peanuts (or any kind of nut) with one part soy milk and process until the mixture reaches your desired consistency. These homemade nut butters have no additives and are more nutritious than commercial varieties. Serve them with Soy Whole Wheat Bread (page 106) for a double dose of soy nutrition.

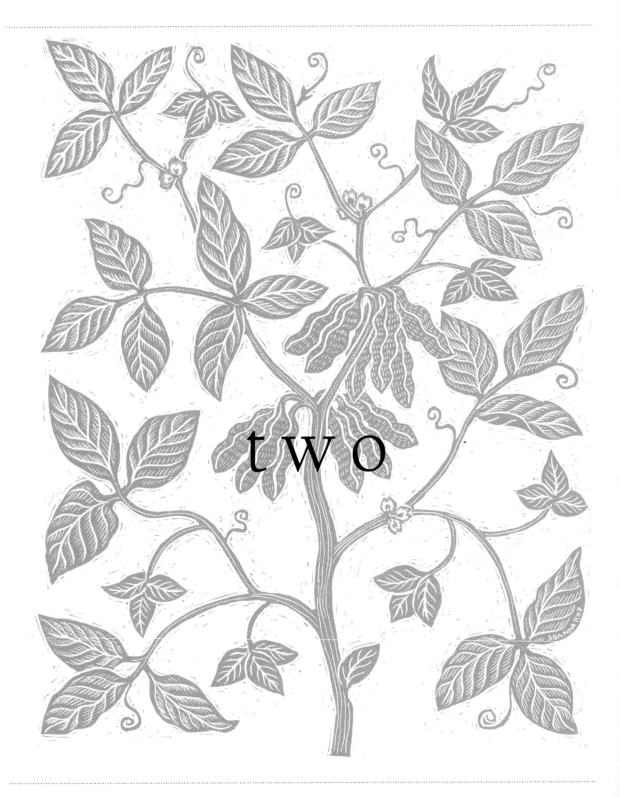

two

salads and vegetables

Cold or hot, soy in all its forms pairs beautifully with vegetables and fruits. In this chapter, you can take your pick of what form of the bean to work with: tofu in Mediterranean Tofu Salad, soy milk in Garlic Mashed Potatoes with Soy Milk, soy yogurt in Curried Eggplant, tempeh in Tempeh Picnic Salad, whole soybeans in Black and White Bean Salad. Fresh fruits and vegetables are marvelous sources of vitamins, minerals, and fiber; with the addition of soy foods, these dishes are also rich in protein and provide all the other benefits of soy.

Salads offer one of the easiest ways to incorporate soy into your diet. Keep some Soy Green Goddess or Mustard Tarragon Soy Vinaigrette handy in the refrigerator to dress your greens. Or toss in flavorful cubes of soy cheese or soy ham: Chef's Salad with Creamy Herb Dressing provides an incredible 29 grams of soy protein per serving. Serve some of the salads in this chapter— such as Tofu Waldorf Salad, Confetti Slaw with Tomato-Soy Yogurt Dressing, or Spinach Salad with Warm Soy Bacon Dressing—as crisp counterpoints to a main course. Others, such as Fall Fruit Salad with Nuts and Tempeh or Soy Tortellini Salad, make great light meals by themselves, with the addition of a slice of warm Soy Olive Bread (page 105) or crusty French bread.

Some of the vegetable dishes in this chapter make great light meals, too. Twice Baked Potatoes—crisp skins stuffed with a mixture of cheese, soy ham, and baked potatoes—can't be beat for a satisfying lunch. Or choose simpler preparations to complement main dishes. I like to serve Creamed Spinach and Garlic Mashed Potatoes with Soy Milk along with Soy Meat Loaf (page 160); Asparagus Spears with Garlic Aïoli is a wonderful accompaniment for Arroz con Tempeh (page 165).

Consider these recipes a starting point for experimentation. You can pair any vegetable you choose with the velvety sauce in the recipe for Broccoli with Soy Mornay Sauce. Mix sweet and Yukon Gold potatoes in the Potatoes au Gratin; serve the Curried Eggplant and Creamed Spinach along with Cucumber Raita (page 46) as part of an Indian buffet. When you combine soy and vegetables, almost anything goes.

Mixed Baby Greens with
Mustard Tarragon Soy Vinaigrette

Tarragon, with its hint of anise flavor, melds perfectly with tangy Dijon mustard in this French-inspired dressing. The soy milk adds creaminess to the vinaigrette, making it cling luxuriously to mixed leafy greens. Many markets sell mesclun, a mixed combination of delicate baby lettuces, or you can make your own mixture with Bibb lettuce, radicchio, watercress, endive, and arugula.

Vinaigrette

½ cup white wine vinegar

2 tablespoons Dijon mustard

½ teaspoon salt

½ teaspoon white pepper

¼ cup chopped parsley

2 teaspoons dried tarragon, plus
   1 sprig of tarragon

1 cup soy milk

2 tablespoons olive oil

Salad

1 pound mixed baby greens,
   washed and spun dry

3 large white mushrooms, thinly
   sliced

3 ounces alfalfa sprouts, for garnish

1. In a food processor or blender, combine the vinegar, mustard, salt, pepper, parsley, tarragon, and soy milk on high speed until pureed.

2. Reduce the speed, and with the motor running, slowly drizzle the oil into the blender, until dressing is emulsified. Set aside while you prepare the greens. (Makes 2 cups; extra dressing will keep in the refrigerator for up to 1 week.)

3. Wash the greens, dry thoroughly, and combine with the mushrooms in a salad bowl. Toss with about ¾ cup of dressing. Sprinkle alfalfa sprouts on top and serve.

SERVES 6

Calories	Total Protein	Soy Protein	Carbohydrate	Fat	Cholesterol	Fiber	Sodium
60.5	3.7 g	0.5 g	8.4 g	2.2 g	0 mg	4 g	131 mg

Information is per serving, including dressing.

Fennel Salad with
Soy Green Goddess Dressing

This is a delicious, unusual salad made with fennel, a crisp, faintly licorice-flavored vegetable. Long popular in Europe, fennel has become widely available in American grocery stores as more people come to appreciate its versatility and lively taste. Look for firm, unbruised, medium bulbs with fresh, celerylike stalks. Fennel is perfectly complemented by this herbal Green Goddess dressing; the creaminess comes from soy milk rather than the sour cream and mayonnaise of a traditional green goddess. Thick and tangy, the dressing also makes a great dip for crudités or sauce for steamed vegetables. Serve the salad as an accompaniment to Grilled Tempeh with Barbecue Sauce (page 154) or Broiled Tofu with Five-Onion Sauce (page 143).

Dressing

10 ounces green peas, fresh or
   frozen
½ cup soy milk
2 tablespoons lemon juice
2 garlic cloves, minced
3 sprigs of mint
6 leaves fresh basil, chopped
Salt and white pepper to taste

Salad

1 fennel bulb, sliced
1 medium cucumber, peeled,
   seeded, and sliced
4 scallions, white and tender green
   parts, chopped
2 cups shredded carrots
1 pound mixed salad greens,
   washed and spun dry

1. In a food processor or blender, puree the peas, soy milk, lemon juice, garlic, mint, basil, salt, and pepper. Chill.
2. Combine the fennel, cucumber, scallions, carrots, and greens in a serving bowl. Pour dressing over and toss lightly. Serve immediately.

SERVES 6

Calories	Total Protein	Soy Protein	Carbohydrate	Fat	Cholesterol	Fiber	Sodium
106.5	6 g	3 g	20 g	0.8 g	0 mg	7 g	90 mg

Information is per serving, including dressing.

Spinach Salad with
Warm Soy Bacon Dressing

Crisp spinach leaves are the perfect foil for the warm, sweet-and-sour dressing for this memorable salad, based on a French classic. Soy bacon stands in for regular bacon, providing rich flavor but little fat and no cholesterol. It's a wonderful starter for a meal of Soy Meat Loaf (page 160) and Garlic Mashed Potatoes with Soy Milk (page 55).

Salad

12 ounces soy bacon strips

1 tablespoon soybean oil

1 12-ounce package cleaned
   spinach leaves (about 6 cups
   loosely packed)

½ cup sliced fresh mushrooms

1 red onion, sliced thinly

Dressing

1 tablespoon olive oil

½ small onion, chopped

½ cup red wine vinegar

½ cup soy milk

2 tablespoons sugar

2 teaspoons cornstarch, dissolved in
   2 tablespoons water

1 teaspoon salt

Pepper to taste

1. Fry the soy bacon in soybean oil 1 minute on each side until crisp, and set aside. Dice when cool.

2. Divide the spinach leaves, mushrooms, and red onion among 6 large salad plates and chill or place in a cool area of the kitchen.

3. Heat the oil in a small saucepan on medium-high heat, and sauté the onion until translucent, about 5 minutes. Add the vinegar, soy milk, and sugar, bring to a boil, and reduce the heat to low.

4. Add the cornstarch, stirring as mixture thickens slightly. Add the diced bacon. Let cool slightly and season with salt and pepper. Pour the warm dressing over salad greens.

SERVES 6

Calories	Total Protein	Soy Protein	Carbohydrate	Fat	Cholesterol	Fiber	Sodium
139	11.5 g	10 g	10 g	2.9 g	0 mg	2.5 g	403 mg

Information is per serving, including dressing.

Soy Caesar Salad with Herbed Croutons

If you've given up Caesar salads because of the raw egg in the traditional dressing, here's a wonderful solution. This egg-free rendition gets its flavor from soy parmesan cheese and plenty of garlic. The dressing keeps well, refrigerated, for up to three days.

Dressing

¼ cup olive oil

¾ cup soy milk

4 garlic cloves, minced

¼ cup soy parmesan cheese

½ teaspoon salt

½ teaspoon black pepper

Salad

1 large head romaine lettuce, rinsed and spun dry

Croutons

2 slices whole wheat bread

1 tablespoon olive oil

1 teaspoon dried oregano

1. In a medium mixing bowl, whisk together the olive oil, soy milk, garlic, soy parmesan cheese, salt, and pepper. (The dressing can be made ahead and refrigerated for up to one week.)

2. Preheat the oven to 450°F.

3. Tear the lettuce into bite-size pieces and chill in a large bowl.

4. Cut the bread into small cubes. Toss the bread with the olive oil and oregano, and place on an ungreased baking sheet. Bake for 10 minutes or until brown. Remove from the oven and set aside.

5. Just before serving, toss the lettuce with the dressing, sprinkling the croutons on top.

SERVES 6

Calories	Total Protein	Soy Protein	Carbohydrate	Fat	Cholesterol	Fiber	Sodium
139	5 g	3 g	8 g	9 g	0 mg	2 g	307 mg

Information is per serving, including dressing.

Warm Salad
of Roasted Portobello Mushrooms
with Creamy Garlic Dressing

Warm salad? You may think it's a contradiction in terms until you try this mellow mushroom dish. Broiling brings out the woodsy flavor of portobello mushrooms, while the cool greens and piquant garlic dressing offer a satisfying contrast in texture and flavor. This makes a great start to a dinner of Soy Cheese Manicotti (page 173).

Dressing

8 garlic cloves

2 tablespoons olive oil, plus a little
  extra for brushing

2 tablespoons honey

3 tablespoons balsamic vinegar

3 tablespoons red wine vinegar

¼ teaspoon salt

⅛ teaspoon pepper

1 cup soy milk

Salad

3 large portobello mushrooms

2 tablespoons olive oil

3 garlic cloves, finely chopped

4 plum tomatoes, chopped

1 head red-leaf lettuce

1. Preheat the oven to 375°F. Peel the garlic and place the cloves on a cookie sheet. Brush lightly with olive oil and roast for 15 minutes, until slightly brown. Remove and cool.

2. Combine the roasted garlic, honey, vinegars, salt, and pepper in a food processor or blender. Blend on high speed for 30 seconds while slowly drizzling the remaining olive oil into the mixture. Gradually add the soy milk and continue blending until the mixture attains a creamy consistency. Set aside. (Makes 1½ cups; extra dressing will keep in the refrigerator for up to 1 week.)

3. Preheat the broiler. Cut the mushrooms into long, thick slices and coat with olive oil. Place in a small shallow, baking pan and sprinkle chopped garlic on top. Cover with the tomatoes and broil for 15 minutes, until tomatoes are soft. Set aside.

4. Line 6 salad plates with lettuce. Divide the mushrooms and tomatoes among them, arranging the slices as evenly as possible. Drizzle 2 tablespoons of dressing over each portion and serve immediately.

Calories	Total Protein	Soy Protein	Carbohydrate	Fat	Cholesterol	Fiber	Sodium
129	2.7 g	1 g	19 g	6 g	0 mg	2 g	57 mg

Information is per serving, including dressing.

Garlic Mashed Potatoes with Soy Milk

Here's the ultimate comfort food—especially because soy milk makes mashed potatoes even more creamy than regular milk does.

 3 large baking potatoes
 1 teaspoon vegetable oil
 6 garlic cloves, finely minced
 ¾ cup soy milk
 3 tablespoons soy margarine
 Chopped parsley, for garnish

1. Peel and dice the potatoes. In a steamer basket set over boiling water, steam the potatoes for 15 minutes, until cubes are soft.

2. While the potatoes are steaming, heat the oil over medium heat in a small saucepan and lightly sauté the garlic, about 30 seconds. Add the soy milk and reduce to a simmer. Continue to cook the mixture while the potatoes finish steaming.

3. When the potatoes are soft, mash them with a potato masher and stir in the soy milk mixture and the margarine, adding just as much as needed to reach the desired consistency. Garnish with parsley and serve.

S E R V E S   6

Calories	Total Protein	Soy Protein	Carbohydrate	Fat	Cholesterol	Fiber	Sodium
168	3 g	3 g	24 g	7 g	0 mg	3 g	11 mg

Information is per serving.

Confetti Slaw with
Tomato-Soy Yogurt Dressing

This colorful salad combines red and green cabbage with carrots and raisins. The tangy yogurt-tomato dressing makes for a spicy twist on traditional cole slaw; it's also much lighter than the usual mayonnaise-based sauce. I like to garnish this with thinly sliced Red Delicious apples for their vibrant color and for their sweetness, which is a perfect complement for cabbage. This salad is a great accompaniment for almost any main course, especially simple ones such as Grilled Tempeh with Barbecue Sauce (page 154) or the Garden Kabobs with Orange Sauce (page 155).

Dressing

2 cups tomato juice

1 small onion, minced

¼ cup chopped parsley

½ green bell pepper, minced

¼ cup chopped chives

3 garlic cloves, minced

1 teaspoon Tabasco sauce

1 tablespoon cornstarch

¾ cup soy yogurt

Salad

½ head green cabbage, shredded

¼ head red cabbage, shredded

2 medium carrots, grated

1 cup seedless raisins

2 medium Red Delicious apples,
 cored, quartered, and sliced thinly

1. Combine the tomato juice, onion, parsley, pepper, chives, garlic, and Tabasco in a saucepan and bring the mixture to a boil. Continue to boil until the liquid is reduced by half, about 10 minutes. Remove from the heat.

2. Sprinkle the cornstarch over the mixture and stir vigorously with a whisk to eliminate any lumps. Transfer the mixture to a food processor or blender container and let cool to room temperature.

3. Add the soy yogurt and puree on high speed until smooth. Chill while assembling the salad ingredients.

4. Divide the green cabbage among 6 salad plates. In the center of the green cabbage, arrange the red cabbage. On top of that, sprinkle the shredded carrots and raisins. Fan the apple slices around the base and serve with the

dressing passed separately. (For more casual meals, the salad and dressing can be tossed together like cole slaw, with the apple slices as garnish.)

SERVES 6

Calories	Total Protein	Soy Protein	Carbohydrate	Fat	Cholesterol	Fiber	Sodium
189	4 g	1 g	40 g	0.5 g	0 mg	9 g	41 mg

Information is per serving, including dressing.

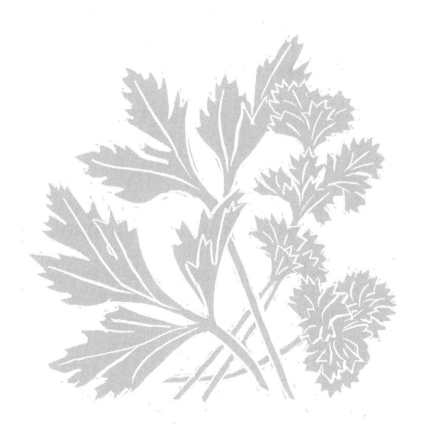

How to Zest Citrus Fruits

Citrus zest—the colorful outer layer of the skin of a citrus fruit—adds strong flavor to dressings, baked goods, and other foods. There are a few tricks to removing the zest properly, however, since the white pith just underneath the zest is very bitter.

One technique is to use a special tool called a zester, which peels away thin ribbons of colored zest and leaves behind the pith. Mince these ribbons finely or leave them intact for decorative garnishes.

Another, simpler way is to use a vegetable peeler and scrape away just the zest carefully, being sure to leave the pith behind. Then mince the zest finely with a sharp knife.

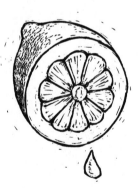

California Fruit Salad with Honey Lemon Yogurt Dressing

Pour this sweet dressing over a fresh fruit salad or use it as a dip for strawberries and cantaloupe spears.

Dressing

1 cup plain soy yogurt
¼ cup soy milk
¼ cup honey
1 tablespoon lemon juice
2 tablespoons chopped fresh mint
Zest of 1 small lemon, minced

Salad

12 ounces soy ham, cut into thin strips
½ small cantaloupe, peeled, seeded, and diced
½ small honeydew melon, peeled, seeded, and diced
¾ pound seedless red grapes
1 head romaine lettuce, torn into bite-size pieces
2 kiwis, peeled and sliced into half-circles

1. Combine the yogurt, soy milk, honey, lemon juice, mint, and lemon zest in a food processor or blender and mix until well combined. Chill until ready to use.

2. In a large salad bowl, toss the ham, cantaloupe, honeydew, and grapes. Gently fold in the dressing until the fruit and ham are coated.

3. Line 6 plates with lettuce and mound the fruit mixture in the middle. Garnish with kiwi slices and serve immediately.

SERVES 6

Calories	Total Protein	Soy Protein	Carbohydrate	Fat	Cholesterol	Fiber	Sodium
269	18.5 g	16.2 g	7 g	1.6 g	0 mg	0 g	389 mg

Information is per serving, including dressing.

Tofu Waldorf Salad

The classic Waldorf salad was created a century ago by the renown Oscar Tschirky at the prestigious Waldorf-Astoria Hotel in New York. This updated version adds cubes of tofu to the traditional combination of apples, walnuts, and celery. Served with warm slices of Pumpernickel Bread (page 107), this makes a substantial and wholesome lunch.

1 cup Tofu Mayonnaise (see sidebar)

1 tablespoon honey

1 pound extra-firm tofu, cut into 1-inch cubes

3 celery stalks, chopped

¼ cup dark raisins

¼ cup golden raisins

3 Red Delicious apples, cored and chopped

1 orange, peeled, sectioned, and cut into chunks

½ cup chopped walnuts

1. Mix the mayonnaise and honey until smooth, using a wire whisk or a blender.
2. Place the tofu, vegetables, fruits, and nuts in a salad bowl and pour the dressing over it. Toss very gently and chill for 45 minutes before serving.

SERVES 6

Calories	Total Protein	Soy Protein	Carbohydrate	Fat	Cholesterol	Fiber	Sodium
307	8 g	6 g	35 g	17 g	10 mg	5 g	224 mg

Information is per serving.

Tofu Mayonnaise

1 pound soft, silken tofu

4 tablespoons apple cider vinegar

1 teaspoon Dijon mustard

½ teaspoon salt

⅔ cup vegetable oil

1 tablespoon lemon juice (optional)

1. In a food processor or blender on medium speed, puree the tofu until smooth. Add the vinegar, mustard, and salt and mix until thoroughly combined.
2. Turn the machine on high and drizzle the oil in slowly until the mixture thickens.
3. Taste for seasonings, adding lemon juice if desired. The mayonnaise will keep in the refrigerator for 2 weeks.

MAKES 2 CUPS

Calories: 44, Total Protein: 1 g.

Soy Protein: 1 g.

Carbohydrate: 0 g, Fat: 4 g.

Cholesterol: 0 mg, Fiber: 0 g.

Sodium: 15 mg

Information for a 2-tablespoon serving.

Mediterranean Tofu Salad

This is very much like a Greek salad, with black olives, ripe tomatoes, crunchy cucumber, and aromatic red onion in a tangy, garlicky vinaigrette. Healthful tofu replaces the traditional feta cheese. Extra-firm tofu is best, as it holds its shape the way feta would. Use good-quality, briny, imported olives.

Salad

1 pound firm tofu, cubed

1 cup garbanzo beans (drained, canned, or cooked and dried)

½ cup black olives, pitted and sliced (preferably Kalamata)

½ cup chopped parsley

½ medium red onion, peeled and sliced in thin matchsticks

3 ripe, medium tomatoes, diced

1 small cucumber, seeded and diced

Dressing

⅓ cup olive oil

2 tablespoons red wine vinegar

2 garlic cloves, minced

1 teaspoon Dijon mustard

2 teaspoons honey

1 tablespoon dried oregano

1 teaspoon cayenne pepper, or to taste

½ teaspoon salt

¼ teaspoon white pepper

1. Place the tofu, beans, olives, parsley, and vegetables in a salad bowl.
2. Whisk together all the dressing ingredients and pour over salad. Toss lightly and serve.

SERVES 6

Calories	Total Protein	Soy Protein	Carbohydrate	Fat	Cholesterol	Fiber	Sodium
263	9 g	6 g	12 g	20 g	0 mg	5 g	577 mg

Information is per serving, including dressing.

South of the Border Tofu Salad

This is just like a Mexican taco salad—minus the beef or chicken. The tofu absorbs the flavor of the cumin and chili for a flavorful kick. Use extra-firm tofu, so the cubes hold their shape as they sauté. The finishing touch of sour cream (soy, in this case) and guacamole are traditional (but optional) accompaniments.

6 6-inch corn tortillas

2 tablespoons vegetable oil

½ cup chopped onion

2 garlic cloves, minced

1 ripe, medium tomato, coarsely
  chopped

1 tablespoon chili powder

1 teaspoon ground cumin

1½ pounds extra-firm tofu, cut into
  1-inch cubes

1 head romaine lettuce, washed,
  spun dry, and shredded

8 ounces soy cheddar cheese,
  shredded

6 tablespoons soy sour cream
  (optional)

6 tablespoons Tofu Guacamole
  (optional, page 37)

1. Preheat the oven to 400°F. Place tortillas in broiler below oven and toast for 2 minutes, then remove and cool.

2. In a medium saucepan, heat the vegetable oil and sauté the onion and garlic until onion is translucent, about 5 minutes.

3. Add the tomato, chili, cumin, and tofu and cook for 8 to 10 minutes.

4. Place a tortilla on each of 6 plates and divide the tofu mixture evenly among the tortillas. Top with shredded lettuce and shredded cheese, and add the soy sour cream and guacamole, if desired. Serve with your favorite salsa.

SERVES 6

Calories	Total Protein	Soy Protein	Carbohydrate	Fat	Cholesterol	Fiber	Sodium
307	24 g	20 g	20 g	16 g	21 mg	5.5 g	256 mg

Information is per serving, without sour cream and guacamole.

Cooking Dried Soybeans

Canned soybeans are a wonderful time-saver. I always keep plenty in my pantry so I can whip up chilies and bean salads in a matter of minutes. But if you have a few hours to spare, it's easy (as well as cheaper) to prepare dried soybeans for use in any recipe calling for cooked soybeans.

First, rinse and pick over the dried beans. Soak them overnight in water to cover. Drain them and place in a large pot with fresh water to cover by a few inches. Bring to a boil, reduce the heat to a simmer, and cook for three hours. You can add an onion and a little salt, if you wish, but because the beans will likely be combined with other ingredients later, it is not necessary to season them. Soybeans, whether cooked in this manner or canned, are firmer than other legumes, so don't fear they are underdone if they still seem al dente.

Black and White Bean Salad

The combination of black beans and white soybeans, plus flecks of red onion and green pepper, makes this a festive salad. It works well as a light lunch or as an addition to a summer barbecue. The soybeans are a little firmer than the black beans and add unexpected texture to this colorful dish.

1 15-ounce can black beans
1 15-ounce can cooked soybeans (or substitute 1 cup dried; see sidebar; both available at health food stores)
½ medium red onion, chopped
1 small green bell pepper, chopped
¼ cup chopped parsley
3 tablespoons olive oil
2 tablespoons red wine vinegar
¼ teaspoon salt
White pepper to taste
Fresh salad greens, for serving

1. Drain the beans and combine them in a large bowl. Add the onion, pepper, and parsley.
2. Sprinkle on the oil, vinegar, salt, and white pepper, and gently toss the salad until thoroughly combined. Chill and serve as an appetizer or side salad, mounded on fresh greens.

SERVES 6

Calories	Total Protein	Soy Protein	Carbohydrate	Fat	Cholesterol	Fiber	Sodium
161	7.5 g	3 g	17 g	8 g	0 mg	2 g	382 mg

Information is per serving.

Fall Fruit Salad
with Nuts and Tempeh

The addition of cubed soy mozzarella and tempeh elevates this fruit salad to a nutritious meal by itself. Slivered almonds and crunchy celery add delicious texture. I serve it accompanied by assorted muffins.

½ cup soy mayonnaise or Tofu
   Mayonnaise (page 59)
1 tablespoon sherry
2 tablespoons white wine vinegar
1 tablespoon honey
1 tablespoon tarragon
1 tablespoon Dijon mustard
8 ounces tempeh

4 ounces soy mozzarella cheese, cut
   into small cubes
½ pound grapes, green and red
1 small red apple, cored and diced
¾ cup slivered almonds, toasted
1 celery stalk, finely chopped
4 scallions, finely chopped, green
   and white parts

1. In a large serving bowl, whisk together the mayonnaise, sherry, vinegar, honey, tarragon, and mustard. Set aside.

2. In a steamer basket set over boiling water, steam the tempeh until soft, about 8 minutes. Let cool and cut into cubes.

3. Add the tempeh, mozzarella, grapes, apples, almonds, celery, and scallions to the serving bowl and toss gently to combine with the dressing. Chill for 1 hour before serving.

SERVES 6

Calories	Total Protein	Soy Protein	Carbohydrate	Fat	Cholesterol	Fiber	Sodium
305	17 g	13 g	27 g	15 g	10 mg	5 g	190 mg

Information is per serving.

Indonesian Tempeh Rice Salad

The famous Indonesian dish known as rijsttafel *consists of a central bowl of steaming rice surrounded by smaller bowls of sweet and savory delicacies—dried fruits, meats, seafood, crunchy vegetables, and nuts—to be mixed in to suit the diner's taste. Inspired by that classic, this is a room-temperature, rice-based salad with an Indonesian flair. Water chestnuts and cashews add crunch; raisins and pineapple add sweetness; and toasted sesame oil and soy sauce add Asian flavor. Nutty-tasting tempeh, which itself is Indonesian in origin, replaces the meats and seafood. You can make this delicious salad a day in advance and serve it the same way you would a substantial pasta salad: as a main course or as an accompaniment to other foods.*

Dressing

⅓ cup peanut oil

3 tablespoons toasted sesame oil

½ cup orange juice

2 garlic cloves, minced

½ teaspoon crushed red pepper

2 tablespoons soy sauce

1 teaspoon salt

1 tablespoon honey

2 tablespoons cider vinegar

1 cup diced pineapple (canned or fresh)

Tempeh mixture

8 ounces tempeh

3 scallions, thinly sliced, green and white parts

1 cup thinly sliced water chestnuts

1 celery stalk, diced

1 medium red bell pepper, diced

1 large carrot, diced

½ cup raisins

½ cup cashews

2 tablespoons sesame seeds

6 cups cooked rice

1. Combine all the dressing ingredients, whisking well, and set aside.

2. Set a steamer basket over boiling water and place the tempeh in it. Steam for about 8 minutes, until tempeh is soft. Remove from heat, let cool until it can be handled, and crumble it into a large salad bowl.

3. Add the vegetables, raisins, nuts, seeds, and rice to the bowl and pour on the dressing. Toss gently to combine. Set aside at room temperature for 1 hour before serving.

Calories	Total Protein	Soy Protein	Carbohydrate	Fat	Cholesterol	Fiber	Sodium
455	12 g	5 g	68 g	15 g	0 mg	4 g	274 mg

Information is per main course serving.

Creamed Spinach

This tangy dish, made with soy yogurt, is a breeze to make. It's the perfect complement to curries, or serve it with Soy Meat Loaf (page 160).

> 3 10-ounce packages frozen chopped spinach
> 3 tablespoons olive oil
> 6 garlic cloves, minced
> 1 teaspoon sesame seeds
> 1½ cups plain soy yogurt

1. Thaw the spinach in a colander. Squeeze out excess juice and set aside.
2. Heat the olive oil in a large saucepan over medium heat and sauté the garlic until slightly browned, about 8 minutes. Add the spinach and sauté until spinach is heated completely through, about 5 minutes.
3. Add the sesame seeds and stir for 1 minute.
4. Add the soy yogurt and mix until the yogurt is heated, about 3 minutes. Serve hot.

SERVES 6

Calories	Total Protein	Soy Protein	Carbohydrate	Fat	Cholesterol	Fiber	Sodium
150	6 g	2 g	17 g	7 g	0 mg	6 g	102 mg

Information is per serving.

Tempeh Picnic Salad

This dish reminds me of chicken salad because of the tempeh's meaty firmness and the sage-scented poultry seasoning in the dressing. In fact, you can use it exactly as you would regular chicken salad: in a sandwich, spread between slices of hearty whole wheat bread and topped with crisp lettuce or sprouts, or as a main course, scooped onto a bed of mixed greens and garnished with cantaloupe spears. It's versatile, simple to prepare, and wonderful for lunch or a light summer supper.

1½ pounds tempeh

½ cup soy mayonnaise or Tofu Mayonnaise (page 59)

4 basil leaves, chopped

½ teaspoon salt

¼ teaspoon white pepper

1 teaspoon poultry seasoning

2 celery stalks, finely chopped

⅓ cup chopped red onion (about ¼ medium red onion)

1. In a large pot, set a steamer basket over boiling water and place the tempeh in it. Steam the tempeh, covered, for 8 minutes or until soft. Remove from the heat and cut the tempeh into ½-inch cubes. Set aside.

2. In medium mixing bowl, whisk together the mayonnaise, basil, salt, pepper, and poultry seasoning. Add the tempeh, celery, and onion and toss gently to combine.

SERVES 6

Calories	Total Protein	Soy Protein	Carbohydrate	Fat	Cholesterol	Fiber	Sodium
334	27 g	26 g	29 g	14 g	0 mg	5 g	292 mg

Information is per serving.

Bombay Tempeh and Lentils

The nuttiness of basmati rice and the spark of curry powder give this room-temperature salad a distinctly Indian panache. Using imported aromatic basmati rice makes all the difference; it is available in the international section of large supermarkets or in specialty markets. The combination of lentils and rice forms the backbone of the Indian diet; the tempeh makes that combination even more nutritious by adding 5 grams of soy protein per serving. Serve as a side dish or as a main course for lunch or dinner. It's especially good accompanied by Chilled Mango Cantaloupe Soy Soup (page 128) or Carrot Ginger Soy Soup (page 123). For a spicier salad, add 1 tablespoon of chili paste to the water when cooking the lentils and split peas.

8 ounces tempeh	1 tablespoon mild curry powder
1½ cups basmati rice	1 garlic clove, minced
½ cup brown lentils	½ cup red lentils
¼ cup green split peas	⅓ cup dried currants
¼ cup yellow split peas	2 scallions, sliced, green and white
1 tablespoon ground ginger	parts

1. Set a steamer basket over boiling water and place the tempeh in it. Steam it, covered, for about 8 minutes, until it is soft. Remove from heat and cool.

2. Cook rice according to package directions and set aside.

3. Bring the brown lentils and green and yellow split peas to a boil in enough water to cover them. Add the ginger, curry powder, and garlic, reduce the heat, and simmer for 45 minutes. Add a little water if necessary to keep mixture moist. Set aside to cool.

4. In a separate pan, cook the red lentils for 15 minutes. Drain and cool.

5. Crumble the tempeh and combine with the lentils, peas, and currants. Garnish with the sliced scallions.

SERVES 6 AS A MAIN COURSE OR 8 AS A SIDE DISH

Calories	Total Protein	Soy Protein	Carbohydrate	Fat	Cholesterol	Fiber	Sodium
206	10 g	5 g	38 g	2 g	0 mg	4 g	5 mg

Information is per main course serving.

Tempeh with Artichokes in a Creamy Tarragon Dressing

Firm, nutty tempeh and baby artichoke hearts are bathed in an anise-scented tarragon dressing. Serve as a dinner salad, accompanying Tofu Spinach Burgers (page 116) or Soy Meat Loaf (page 160), or by itself for lunch, with warm slices of Soy Olive Bread (page 105).

 1 pound tempeh
 ⅔ cup soy mayonnaise or Tofu Mayonnaise (page 59)
 4 tablespoons Dijon mustard
 4 tablespoons olive oil
 2 teaspoons dried tarragon
 ¼ cup finely chopped parsley
 14-ounce can water-packed artichoke hearts,
 drained and cut into quarters
 6 cups mixed greens (optional)

1. Set a steamer basket over boiling water and steam the tempeh until it is soft, about 5 minutes. Let cool and cut into small dices.
2. Blend the mayonnaise, mustard, oil, and tarragon until smooth.
3. Combine the tempeh, parsley, and artichoke hearts in a large bowl. Pour the mayonnaise mixture over all, tossing lightly.
4. Refrigerate for at least 1 hour. Serve on a bed of fresh greens, if desired.

SERVES 6

Calories	Total Protein	Soy Protein	Carbohydrate	Fat	Cholesterol	Fiber	Sodium
349	16 g	14 g	22 g	20 g	7 mg	3 g	261 mg

Information is per serving, including greens.

Caribbean Tempeh Salad

Caribbean cuisine, with its African influences, often features sweet potatoes. This island-style, room-temperature salad combines them with juicy mango and crisp jicama. The tempeh adds texture and substantial soy protein to the dish; the colorful topping of red and green salsa balances the sweetness. This tropical potato salad makes a satisfying summer lunch on its own or is a good companion to grilled foods.

> 2 large sweet potatoes, peeled and cubed
> 1½ pounds tempeh, cubed
> 2 scallions, minced, green and white parts
> 1 small jicama, peeled and cubed
> 1 mango, peeled, seeded, and cubed
> 1 small head romaine lettuce, shredded
> ½ cup medium-spicy chunky red salsa
> ½ cup medium-spicy chunky green salsa

1. In a steamer basket set over boiling water, steam the sweet potato and tempeh cubes until potatoes are tender, about 10 minutes. Set aside to cool.

2. Combine the scallions, jicama, mango, sweet potatoes, and tempeh in a large bowl, and toss gently.

3. Line 6 plates with lettuce and top with the tempeh mixture. Drizzle red salsa and green salsa alternately on each salad and serve immediately. (The tempeh mixture may be made ahead and refrigerated overnight; bring to room temperature before assembling.)

SERVES 6

Calories	Total Protein	Soy Protein	Carbohydrate	Fat	Cholesterol	Fiber	Sodium
331	24 g	24 g	44 g	9.5 g	0 mg	75 g	164 mg

Information is per serving.

Broccoli Tempeh Salad

This substantial salad features crisp broccoli florets and chewy tempeh, flecked with walnuts, raisins, and red onion for contrast. The zingy sweet-and-sour dressing is the perfect complement. For a hearty lunch, serve it with toasted Soy Herb Bread (page 104).

8 ounces tempeh

2 stalks broccoli, cut into bite-size pieces

½ cup soy mayonnaise or Tofu Mayonnaise (page 59)

⅓ cup honey

3 tablespoons cider vinegar

½ cup chopped walnuts

½ cup dark raisins

¼ small red onion, cut into thin matchsticks

Salt and white pepper to taste

Mixed greens

1. In a steamer basket set over boiling water, steam the tempeh and broccoli for 5 minutes, until soft. Remove from the heat and cut into ½-inch cubes.

2. In medium mixing bowl, thoroughly mix the mayonnaise, honey, and vinegar. Add the tempeh, broccoli, walnuts, raisins, and red onion and combine well. Season with salt and pepper and refrigerate for 1 hour or overnight.

3. Serve over a bed of mixed greens.

SERVES 6

Calories	Total Protein	Soy Protein	Carbohydrate	Fat	Cholesterol	Fiber	Sodium
294	10 g	7 g	39 g	13 g	0 mg	5 g	117 mg

Information is per serving.

Soy Tortellini Salad

A colorful mixture of diced vegetables and plump, soy-cheese–filled tortellini, this versatile pasta salad is a delicious way to incorporate soy in your diet. The crisp, garlicky vinaigrette brings out the best in the cheesy pasta. Soy-filled tortellini are available in health food stores; because they freeze well, it's easy to keep some on hand for whipping up dishes such as this one. Serve this just as you would any hearty pasta salad—as a side dish for a casual meal or as a delicious lunch or light supper on its own.

Dressing

½ cup olive oil

3 tablespoons red wine vinegar

2 garlic cloves, minced

½ teaspoon dried oregano

½ teaspoon dried rosemary

¼ teaspoon salt

⅛ teaspoon black pepper

Salad

2 15-ounce packages soy cheese tortellini (available in health food stores)

½ cup cooked peas, fresh or frozen

1 large carrot, diced

1 medium red bell pepper, diced

¼ cup chopped parsley

1. In a large mixing bowl, combine the dressing ingredients and set aside.
2. Cook the tortellini according to package directions and cool completely.
3. Add the tortellini, peas, carrot, and red pepper to the bowl with the dressing. Toss gently to combine and garnish with parsley.

SERVES 6

Calories	Total Protein	Soy Protein	Carbohydrate	Fat	Cholesterol	Fiber	Sodium
456	11 g	10 g	58 g	18 g	0 mg	3 g	534 mg

Information is per serving.

Chef's Salad with Creamy Herb Dressing

With its decoratively arranged sliced vegetables, soy cheeses, and "meats" this satis-fying salad is as fabulous to look at, as it is to eat. And it's a major source of soy protein: 29 grams per serving! Of course, chef's salads are endlessly flexible; you can easily substitute broccoli florets for zucchini, or avocado for squash, or soy bacon for soy turkey, if that's what you have on hand. The fresh-flavored creamy dressing enhances whatever vegetables and "meats" you choose. This dressing is also delicious tossed over a salad of tomatoes and cucumbers, or served as a dip with raw vegetables or focaccia.

Creamy Herb Dressing

½ cup chopped parsley

4 sprigs of basil

2 scallions, chopped, green and white parts

3 garlic cloves, peeled

½ cup soy milk

1 tablespoon honey

1 teaspoon dried thyme

1 teaspoon dried marjoram

1 teaspoon dried dill weed

1 cup vegetable oil

Salad

1 head green or red-leaf lettuce, leaves washed and left whole

1 head romaine lettuce, leaves washed and torn into bite-size pieces

2 large bunches fresh spinach, washed, stems removed, torn into bite-size pieces

1 medium zucchini, cut into 1½-inch matchsticks

1 medium yellow squash, cut into 1½-inch matchsticks

1 medium carrot, cut into 1½-inch matchsticks

6 ounces soy mozzarella cheese, cubed

6 ounces soy cheddar cheese, cubed

6 ounces soy ham or pepperoni, diced

6 ounces soy turkey, diced

6 plum tomatoes, cut into 4 wedges each

1 large cucumber, sliced thinly

½ cup pitted black olives

1. In a food processor or blender, combine the parsley, basil, scallions, and garlic with the soy milk and honey. Blend on high speed until pureed.

2. Lower the speed, add the dried herbs, and with the motor running, slowly drizzle oil into the blender or processor until dressing is emulsified. Set aside. (Makes 2 cups; extra dressing can be stored, refrigerated, for 2 weeks.)

3. Line a large bowl or 6 individual salad bowls with the whole lettuce leaves. Place a bed of romaine and spinach leaves on top.

4. Arrange the zucchini, squash, and carrot sticks decoratively around the outside of the plate. Arrange the soy cheeses and soy meats in alternate rows in the center of the plates. Garnish with tomato wedges, sliced cucumber, and olives.

5. Drizzle about 2 tablespoons of dressing over each salad or pass separately at serving time.

SERVES 6

Calories	Total Protein	Soy Protein	Carbohydrate	Fat	Cholesterol	Fiber	Sodium
339	32.8 g	29 g	20 g	15.6 g	0 mg	6.5 g	960 mg

Information is per serving, including dressing.

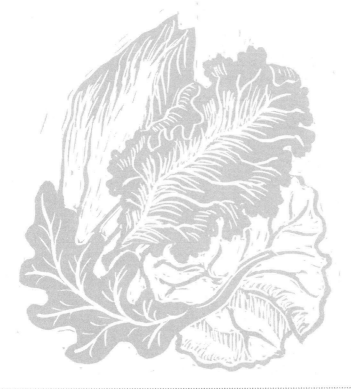

Asparagus Spears with Garlic Aïoli

In the south of France, aïoli—a rich, creamy garlic mayonnaise—is served over all manner of vegetables, both hot and cold, as well as fish, chicken breasts, and meats. Here, it gilds asparagus spears, cooked until just tender. Try this as a delicious accompaniment to Spinach Tempeh in Pastry Pockets (page 156) or Soy Meat Loaf (page 160). This version of aïoli uses Tofu Mayonnaise and doesn't skimp on the garlicky, Provençal flavor. Serve aïoli with other steamed or grilled vegetables, as a dip for raw vegetables, or slathered on slabs of Soy Olive Bread (page 105). For the best consistency, make the aïoli as close as possible to when you'll be serving it.

Aïoli

1 cup plain soy yogurt
⅓ cup soy mayonnaise or Tofu Mayonnaise (page 59)
2 garlic cloves, minced
½ teaspoon dried thyme
½ teaspoon dried oregano
½ teaspoon dried rosemary

2 pounds medium asparagus spears

1. Using a wire whisk, thoroughly combine the yogurt, mayonnaise, garlic, thyme, oregano, and rosemary. Set aside about ¾ cup at room temperature. (Makes 1½ cups; extra dressing may be stored in refrigerator for up to 2 weeks.)

2. Steam the asparagus spears until tender but still bright green and crisp. Serve at once on warm plates, with about 2 tablespoons of aïoli drizzled over each serving.

SERVES 6

Calories	Total Protein	Soy Protein	Carbohydrate	Fat	Cholesterol	Fiber	Sodium
62	4 g	1 g	10 g	1 g	0 mg	1 g	14 mg

Information is per serving, including aïoli.

Corn in Creamy Béchamel Sauce

Digging into a mouthwatering mound of sweet corn kernels bathed in a buttery sauce, wouldn't it be nice to know that what you're eating is actually good for you? Well, when the buttery sauce is Soy Béchamel, it is. Soy milk replaces its dairy counterpart in this thick sauce, adding healthful soy protein. You can also use this béchamel to create creamy masterpieces with spinach, mushrooms, or baby onions. Cover steamed cauliflower with it, sprinkle seasoned bread crumbs on top, and run it under the broiler for a quick gratin. Bind together fillings for crepes, as in Woodland Wild Mushroom Crepes (page 92).

Soy Béchamel Sauce

3 tablespoons soy margarine

¼ cup unbleached all-purpose flour

2½ cups soy milk, at room temperature

2 10-ounce packages frozen corn

1. In a saucepan over medium heat, melt the soy margarine, letting it bubble.
2. Add the flour gradually, constantly stirring. Cook for about 3 minutes, until the mixture reaches a pale yellow color. Slowly stir in the soy milk.
3. Stir constantly while bringing to a boil, 2 to 3 minutes, and remove from the heat. Reserve 1 cup for the creamed corn and keep warm. (Makes about 2½ cups; refrigerate or freeze the rest for another purpose.)
4. Steam the corn until just tender, about 5 mintues. Fold it into the hot sauce and serve immediately.

SERVES 6

Calories	Total Protein	Soy Protein	Carbohydrate	Fat	Cholesterol	Fiber	Sodium
139	5 g	1.6 g	22 g	4 g	0 mg	2.5 g	13 mg

Information is per serving, including sauce.

Broccoli with Soy Mornay Sauce

Broccoli is a workhorse of a vegetable; it's available year-round and it's crammed with vitamins, minerals, and antioxidants. Because it is so useful, however, it suffers a little from overexposure. So blanketing broccoli with this cheesy Soy Mornay Sauce makes it deliciously out of the ordinary—and even healthier. This easy-to-make sauce is an essential to have on hand. Use it to enhance asparagus, cauliflower, Brussels sprouts, spinach, and other vegetables, or to top crepes, poached eggs, or fish dishes. You can make an amazing macaroni and cheese with mornay sauce: just substitute soy cheddar for the jack before combining with cooked elbow noodles and baking.

Mornay Sauce

3 tablespoons soy margarine

¼ cup unbleached all-purpose flour

2½ cups soy milk, at room temperature

¾ cup grated soy jack cheese (about 6 ounces)

2 pounds broccoli

1. In a saucepan over medium heat, melt the soy margarine, letting it bubble.
2. Add the flour gradually, stirring constantly until the mixture reaches a pale yellow color, about 3 minutes. Slowly stir in the soy milk. Stir constantly while bringing to a boil, 2 to 3 minutes, and reduce to a simmer.
3. Add the soy cheese and stir for 3 to 4 minutes as it melts.
4. Remove from the heat. Reserve 1 cup sauce for the broccoli. (Makes about 3 cups; refrigerate the rest for later use.)
5. Trim the broccoli, discarding tough ends. Steam until just tender, about 5 minutes, then remove to a warm serving bowl and pour 1 cup of sauce over it. Serve immediately.

SERVES 6

Calories	Total Protein	Soy Protein	Carbohydrate	Fat	Cholesterol	Fiber	Sodium
147	11 g	6 g	12 g	8 g	0 mg	6 g	264 mg

Information is per serving, including sauce.

Braised Red Cabbage

Cabbage, bursting with vitamins, minerals, and antioxidants, is a healthful food. In this dish, it's also a savory food. The tangy sweet-and-sour sauce, studded with vibrant caraway seeds, bathes the lightly cooked red cabbage—a little like a warm slaw. The soy bacon adds hearty flavor and the goodness of soy to the dish. This goes well with an autumnal main course such as Soy Hungarian Goulash (page 159).

1½ pounds red cabbage
1 tablespoon vegetable oil
3 ounces soy bacon, diced
½ small onion, chopped
1 teaspoon honey
1 teaspoon caraway seeds
½ cup Vegetable Stock (page 120)
3 tablespoons apple cider vinegar
3 tablespoons red wine vinegar
Salt and pepper to taste

1. Cut the cabbage in half and remove the core. Discard any brownish outer leaves. Slice the cabbage into long shreds, but do not chop it. Set aside.
2. Heat the oil in a large skillet over high heat and sauté the soy bacon and onion for 2 minutes. Add the honey and sauté for 1 more minute.
3. Lower the heat and add caraway seeds, cabbage, and stock. Simmer for 20 minutes. Add the vinegars and simmer for 10 more minutes. Season to taste with salt and pepper. Serve immediately.

SERVES 6

Calories	Total Protein	Soy Protein	Carbohydrate	Fat	Cholesterol	Fiber	Sodium
90	4 g	3 g	9 g	2.6 g	0 mg	1 g	106 mg

Information is per serving.

Curried Eggplant

Eggplant makes a wonderful canvas for almost any kind of seasoning, which is why it is beloved in so many great cuisines, from French to Italian to Chinese. Here, in an Indian-inspired dish, cubes of eggplant are steamed until just tender and then lightly simmered with a heady mixture of curry, cumin, ginger, and garlic. Tangy soy yogurt adds creaminess and the benefits of soy to this spicy side dish. It goes perfectly with other Indian recipes, such as Bombay Tempeh and Lentils (page 67).

2 teaspoons ground cumin

1 teaspoon cayenne pepper

2 tablespoons curry powder

¼ cup water

2 medium eggplants, peeled and cut
  into 1-inch cubes

1 tablespoon vegetable oil

1 large onion, chopped

6 garlic cloves, minced

1 1-inch piece fresh ginger, minced

8 plum tomatoes, diced

½ cup plain soy yogurt

Salt and black pepper to taste

1. Put the cumin, cayenne, and curry powder in the water to steep while preparing the rest of the ingredients.

2. Set a steamer basket over boiling water and steam the eggplant cubes for 10 minutes, until soft. Set aside.

3. Over high heat, in a large sauté pan, heat the oil and sauté the onion until slightly browned, approximately 8 minutes. Add the garlic and ginger, sautéing another 30 seconds.

4. Add the eggplant, tomatoes, and seasoning mixture and simmer for 5 minutes. Stir in the yogurt and simmer for 10 more minutes. Add salt and pepper to taste. Serve warm, or refrigerate for up to 2 days and serve chilled.

SERVES 6

Calories	Total Protein	Soy Protein	Carbohydrate	Fat	Cholesterol	Fiber	Sodium
108	3 g	1 g	18 g	3 g	0 mg	1 g	32 mg

Information is per serving.

Broiled Tomato Parmesan Slices

Slice ripe tomatoes in half, sprinkle on a cheesy bread-crumb topping, and brown them under a hot broiler for a delicious, no-fuss side dish. They add a splash of color to whatever you serve them with, and are especially good with Spinach Tempeh in Pastry Pockets (page 156).

⅓ cup olive oil
⅓ cup soy parmesan cheese
¾ cup bread crumbs
2 tablespoons chopped parsley
6 whole medium tomatoes

1. Preheat the broiler.
2. In a medium bowl, combine the olive oil, soy cheese, bread crumbs, and parsley, and mix thoroughly. Slice off the ends of each tomato and cut in half. Broil the tomatoes for 3 minutes. Remove from the broiler and leave in pan.
3. Sprinkle the crumb mixture evenly over the tomato halves and return them to the broiler. Broil for 2 more minutes and serve immediately.

SERVES 6

Calories	Total Protein	Soy Protein	Carbohydrate	Fat	Cholesterol	Fiber	Sodium
166	4 g	2 g	9 g	12.5 g	0 mg	2.6 g	48 mg

Information is for 2 tomato halves, including topping.

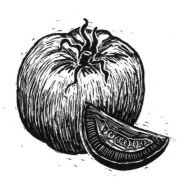

Twice-Baked Potatoes

Crisp potato skins heaped with creamy, bacon-flecked mashed potatoes and melted cheese . . . yum. This wonderfully satisfying dish makes a good light lunch or supper, served with a bowl of steaming Soybean Minestrone (page 127). If you don't have soy bacon on hand, vary the recipe by topping the potato with steamed broccoli florets, then cover with grated cheese.

> 6 baking potatoes
> 6 ounces soy bacon
> ¼ cup soy milk
> 1 ounce soy cheddar cheese, shredded
> ⅔ cup soy sour cream
> 1 tablespoon chopped chives

1. Preheat the oven to 400°F. Scrub the potatoes well, leaving the skins on. Place potatoes in a baking pan and bake for 1 hour. Reduce the oven temperature to 350°F.

2. In a medium skillet, sauté the soy bacon and set aside. When the potatoes are done, remove from the oven and set aside until they are cool enough to handle.

3. Cut a ½-inch slice off the potatoes lengthwise and scoop out the pulp, leaving enough to hold the skin together. In a large bowl, using a wire whip or potato masher, mix the soy bacon and soy milk together with the pulp until combined.

4. Refill each potato skin with the mixture, and cover each with a sprinkling of soy cheddar cheese. Bake for 5 to 8 minutes. Serve with sour cream and chives on the side.

SERVES 6

Calories	Total Protein	Soy Protein	Carbohydrate	Fat	Cholesterol	Fiber	Sodium
358	15 g	10 g	53 g	8 g	0 mg	6 g	348 mg

Information is for 1 potato, not including topping.

Potatoes au Gratin

A mouthwatering golden-brown crust of cheese and toasted bread crumbs cloaks tender slices of potato in this soy adaptation of an old favorite. The potatoes absorb the creamy soy milk as they bake, giving them rich flavor and the benefits of soy protein. Serve this with Tempeh Dijonaisse (page 153) or Grilled Tempeh with Barbecue Sauce (page 154).

4 baking potatoes, peeled but left whole
½ cup soy milk
4 ounces soy jack cheese, finely grated
¼ cup bread crumbs

1. Place the potatoes in a steamer basket over boiling water and cover. Steam for 15 minutes, until soft. Remove from heat.
2. Preheat the oven to 350°F. Transfer the potatoes to a cutting board and gently slice each potato into ¼-inch pieces. Place into a slightly greased 8 by 8-inch baking pan and cover with the soy milk. Top with the soy jack cheese and bread crumbs. Bake for 20 minutes or until bread crumbs are browned.

SERVES 6

Calories	Total Protein	Soy Protein	Carbohydrate	Fat	Cholesterol	Fiber	Sodium
204	8 g	5 g	35 g	4 g	0 mg	4 g	145 mg

Information is per serving.

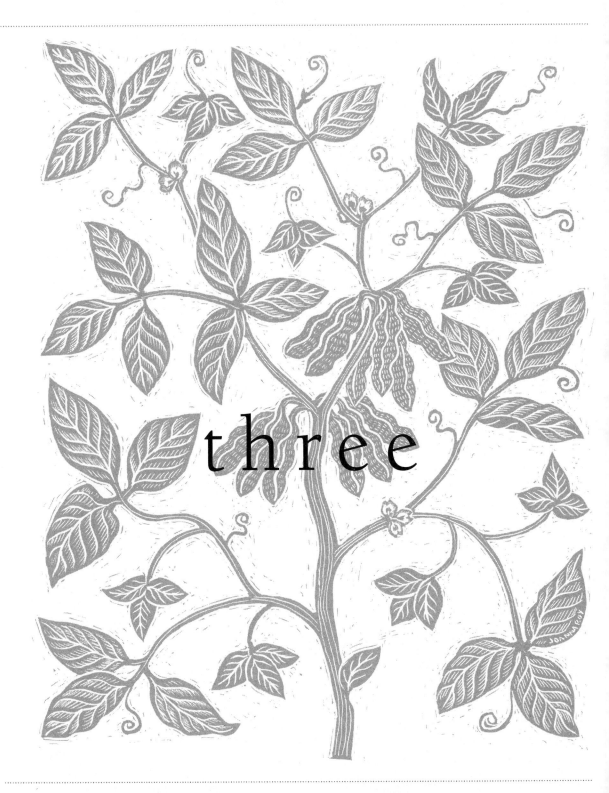

three

brunch and breads

There's nothing nicer than a cozy Sunday brunch or breakfast: fresh coffee or tea, family and friends (or just the newspaper), and soul-satisfying foods hot from the oven. The only problem is that the traditional brunch foods we love, such as eggs and baked goods, tend to be the heaviest in fat and cholesterol.

Well, you'll never miss the eggs at one of my brunches. Here are soy-based quiches as delectable as the cholesterol-laden originals; pancakes and crepes light as feathers; biscuits and scones; even scrambled "eggs"—tofu sautéed with peppers and onions that's every bit as satisfying as the heartiest coffee-shop special. Once you've mastered the basics, it's easy to vary crepe fillings or quiche ingredients to suit individual tastes. Brunches starring soy products have another advantage, too. Unlike eggs, which tend to toughen when kept warm over low heat, soy dishes can be warmed without harm, making brunch or breakfast a lot less pressured.

Nothing is more appealing—at brunch, breakfast, or any other time of the day—than the scent of homemade breads and muffins filling the air. Adding soy to baked goods makes giving into temptation a lot healthier—and just as delicious. As you will see, nothing could be easier than baking with soy. The following recipes for quick breads, muffins, and yeast breads use soy products instead of eggs, milk, and butter. There are a few basic rules for substitution that allow a cook to adapt many bread recipes. Generally, 6 ounces of tofu equals one whole egg, and 1 cup of soy milk equals 1 cup of cow's milk. Egg replacer, which has soy as an ingredient, can be used according to package directions in place of eggs. Soy quick breads and muffins made without eggs will be moister and have a denser texture than those made with eggs. Yeast breads generally turn out very similar to their soy-free originals. Most of these recipes call for all-purpose or whole wheat flour.

You'll find a range of recipes in this chapter, from the sweet to the savory. Soy Cheese Corn Bread, for example, uses soy milk and soy cheddar to produce a moist and cheesy complement to any chili or stew. Soy Sour Cream Lemon Loaf gets its dense richness from soy sour cream as well as soy milk. Soy Whole Wheat Bread uses soy milk and soy flour to make the perfect sandwich bread. They're all sure to become family favorites.

Soy Nut Granola

This fruity, crunchy granola is substantially lower in fat than most commercial varieties—and offers the extra bonus of soy protein. Serve it with cold soy milk or as a topping for soy yogurt or soy-based frozen desserts. It will keep up to two weeks, refrigerated in an airtight container.

1 cup honey

1 tablespoon vegetable oil

1½ teaspoons vanilla extract

6 cups old-fashioned or quick-cooking rolled oats
   (not instant)

1 cup soy nuts

1 cup wheat germ

1 cup oat bran

3 cups coarsely chopped assorted pitted, dried fruit,
    such as apples, apricots, pineapple, raisins, dates,
    cranberries, papaya, or mango

1. Preheat the oven to 350°F. and line 2 baking sheets with parchment paper.

2. In a large mixing bowl, with a wire whip, whisk the honey, oil, and vanilla together until thoroughly combined. Add the rolled oats, soy nuts, wheat germ, and oat bran, mixing well.

3. Spread the mixture on the baking sheets and bake for 20 minutes, until golden brown. Remove from oven. When the mixture has cooled completely, add the dried fruits. Store in an airtight container.

MAKES 48 OUNCES

Calories	Total Protein	Soy Protein	Carbohydrate	Fat	Cholesterol	Fiber	Sodium
372	15 g	12 g	65 g	7.6 g	0 mg	11 g	3.5 mg

Information is for a 4-ounce portion.

Soy Milk Pancakes

If you like flapjacks, I guarantee you won't be able to taste the difference in this healthier version. They cook more quickly than traditional pancakes, though, so watch them carefully to prevent burning.

1 cup unbleached all-purpose flour
½ tablespoon sugar
1 tablespoon baking powder
½ teaspoon salt
½ teaspoon baking soda
1½ cups soy milk
1 tablespoon vegetable oil
¼ cup fresh berries (optional)
Syrup, honey, or preserves for topping, as desired

1. In a medium mixing bowl, sift together the flour, sugar, baking powder, salt, and baking soda.

2. In a large bowl, beat together the soy milk and oil.

3. Gradually add the flour mixture to the soy milk mixture, beating after each addition to make a smooth, thin batter. Fold in the berries at this point, if using.

4. Spray a large nonstick pan with cooking spray or lightly grease a large griddle. Heat over medium-high heat until water drops dance on the surface.

5. Pour ¼ cup of batter for each pancake onto the griddle or into the pan and cook until bubbles form, about 1 minute. Turn and cook 30 seconds more. Serve hot, with topping of choice.

MAKES 12 PANCAKES

Calories	Total Protein	Soy Protein	Carbohydrate	Fat	Cholesterol	Fiber	Sodium
54	2.2 g	0.5 g	7.5 g	2 g	0 mg	0.5 g	209 mg

Information is for 1 pancake.

Tomato Chutney

3 medium tomatoes,
   chopped
1 small red onion, chopped
⅓ cup apple cider vinegar
⅓ cup light brown sugar
½ cup light corn syrup
1 tablespoon tomato paste
2½ teaspoons salt
¼ teaspoon white pepper
½ teaspoon ground
   cinnamon
⅛ teaspoon ground cloves
¼ teaspoon ground ginger
6 sprigs of mint, chopped

1. In a medium saucepan over high heat, combine all the ingredients, stirring well. Bring the mixture to a boil, lower the heat to a simmer, cover, and cook until the liquid is reduced to a syrupy consistency, about 45 minutes.
2. Remove pan from the heat and transfer contents to a bowl to cool. Serve at room temperature. The chutney may be made ahead and keeps for up to 2 weeks in the refrigerator.

MAKES 1 CUP

Calories: 70, Total Protein: 0.5 g,

Soy Protein: 0 g,

Carbohydrate: 18 g, Fat: 0 g,

Cholesterol: 0 mg, Fiber: 1 g,

Sodium: 680 mg

Curried Tofu with Red Peppers and Onions

This protein-rich tofu sauté has a texture remarkably similar to scrambled eggs, which makes it a delicious and healthy breakfast alternative. A dab of sweet and spicy Tomato Chutney on the side (see sidebar) makes the curry even zestier. For a special brunch, try it as a filling for Soy Crepes (page 90). The curry, onion, and pepper lend the tofu flavor; for a Mexican variation, replace the curry with a teaspoon each of oregano, cumin, and chili powder.

> 1 tablespoon vegetable oil
> ½ small onion, chopped
> ½ large red bell pepper, chopped
> 1 tablespoon curry powder
> 3 pounds low-fat silken tofu
> Toast or bagels, as accompaniments

1. In a large saucepan, heat the oil over medium-high heat. Add the onion and red bell pepper and sauté, stirring, until onion is translucent, about 5 minutes.
2. Stir in the curry powder.
3. Dice the tofu into ½-inch cubes and add to the saucepan. Cook, stirring gently so as not to break up the tofu, until it is hot, about 5 minutes. Serve immediately, with warm toast or bagels.

SERVES 6

Calories	Total Protein	Soy Protein	Carbohydrate	Fat	Cholesterol	Fiber	Sodium
199	19 g	18 g	7 g	12 g	0 mg	3 g	16 mg

Information is per serving, not including toast or bagels.

Cream Scones

Scones are simple, slightly sweet biscuits. The traditional fare for an English afternoon tea, they also make a great brunch alternative to muffins. In my version, the soy milk and tofu make them healthful while playing up the usual light, flaky texture. The basic scone has a delicate, lemony taste, and you can easily vary flavors. For a crunchy scone, add 2 tablespoons of poppy seeds; for a festive, fruity scone, replace the lemon peel with ½ cup of red currants. Serve scones with jam or honey, if desired.

2 cups unbleached all-purpose flour
½ cup sugar
1 tablespoon baking powder
1 teaspoon salt
½ cup soy margarine, chilled

6 ounces soft tofu
⅓ cup soy milk
2 teaspoons vanilla extract
Zest of 1 large lemon

1. Preheat the oven to 400°F.
2. In a large mixing bowl, combine the flour, sugar, baking powder, and salt.
3. Cut the margarine into small cubes. Using your fingers or 2 sharp knives, mix or cut the margarine into the dry ingredients until it resembles coarse crumbs.
4. In a food processor or blender, combine the tofu, soy milk, and vanilla, pulsing until smooth. The mixture should have the consistency of yogurt. Pour this mixture into the flour mixture, stirring to combine thoroughly. Fold in the lemon zest.
5. On a lightly floured surface, roll the dough out to a ½-inch thickness. Cut into 3-inch rounds with a biscuit cutter and place the rounds on a greased or parchment-lined cookie sheet.
6. Bake for 15 minutes, or until slightly browned. Remove from oven and let cool completely before serving.

MAKES 8 SCONES

Calories	Total Protein	Soy Protein	Carbohydrate	Fat	Cholesterol	Fiber	Sodium
217	5 g	2 g	37 g	5 g	0 mg	1 g	395 mg

Information is for 1 scone.

Tofu, Spinach, and Soy Ham Quiche

Smooth tofu replaces cholesterol-laden eggs in this quiche, but the rich texture remains the same. Starring the classic duo of spinach and (soy) ham, this brunch favorite has a wonderful, rich flavor. Because quiches are such fabulous blank canvases, feel free to experiment with other additions, such as tomatoes and fresh basil or sautéed mushrooms and shallots.

14 ounces soft tofu

1 tablespoon vegetable oil

½ small onion, chopped

2 garlic cloves, minced

3 ounces soy ham, diced

1 10-ounce package frozen chopped
   spinach, thawed and drained

1 teaspoon sea salt

1 9-inch Pie Crust (page 201) or
   commercial pie crust

¼ cup grated soy mozzarella cheese

1. Preheat the oven to 350°F. In a food processor or blender, puree the tofu until smooth.

2. In a large saucepan, heat the oil over medium-high heat. Add the onion and garlic, sautéing until the onion is translucent, about 5 minutes. Add the soy ham and cook another 5 minutes.

3. Stir in the spinach and simmer for 2 to 3 minutes. Remove from heat.

4. Pour the tofu and salt into the spinach mixture, combining well.

5. Spread the mixture evenly in the pie crust. Sprinkle the grated cheese on top and bake for 35 minutes, until browned. Serve hot.

SERVES 6

Calories	Total Protein	Soy Protein	Carbohydrate	Fat	Cholesterol	Fiber	Sodium
144	12 g	11 g	17 g	16 g	0 mg	2 g	762 mg

Information is per serving.

Tofu Florentine

This sauté of tofu, spinach, and mushrooms is a wonderfully versatile dish. It makes a hearty brunch or lunch dish when served with French bread or muffins. Or use it as a filling for crepes (page 90). Or you can make a spicy, south-of-the-border variation by adding a teaspoon of chili powder, wrapping the mixture in a corn tortilla, and topping it with salsa.

> 2 tablespoons olive oil
> 6 large white mushrooms, thinly sliced
> 12 ounces fresh spinach, washed and spun dry
>   (1 package washed salad spinach)
> 2 pounds firm tofu, crumbled
> Salt and pepper to taste

1. In a large sauté pan, heat the oil over medium heat. Add the mushrooms and sauté until soft, about 5 minutes. Add the spinach and cook until completely wilted.

2. Add the crumbled tofu and stir until heated through. Season with salt and pepper and serve at once.

SERVES 6

Calories	Total Protein	Soy Protein	Carbohydrate	Fat	Cholesterol	Fiber	Sodium
164	13 g	13 g	6 g	11 g	0 mg	35 g	112 mg

Information is per serving.

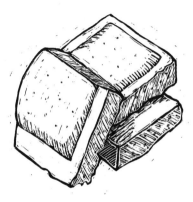

Making Crepes

If you're like most people, the first few crepes in every batch tend to be undercooked, burned, or ragged. Then, as you get the hang of the timing and temperature, the rest look as good as any French chef's. The batter recipes in this book are sufficient to produce 16 crepes, though most dishes using crepes call for only 12. That way, even if the first few are rejects, you'll still have as many as you need. On the other hand, if you manage to produce 16 perfect crepes, congratulate yourself, wrap up the extras, and freeze them for future use.

Soy Crepes

Ah, crepes—those rich-tasting gossamer pancakes stuffed with delicious sweet or savory fillings. I swear you won't be able to tell the difference in taste or texture between my healthful soy version and the original. You can make these crepes ahead of time, since they keep beautifully in the freezer (in freezer bags with waxed paper or parchment between each one).

2 cups whole wheat pastry flour
½ teaspoon salt
2 tablespoons egg replacer
1 cup water

2 cups whole soy milk
2 tablespoons vegetable oil, plus a little for greasing pan

1. Measure the flour and salt into a medium bowl and set aside.
2. In a food processor or blender, combine the egg replacer and water and blend until well mixed. Add the soy milk and oil and process briefly until thoroughly combined.
3. Add the flour mixture a cup at a time, pulsing between additions until smooth.
4. Place a crepe pan over medium heat. Lightly brush entire surface of pan with oil. Lower heat, leaving pan on low heat for about 3 minutes.
5. Lift the pan off the heat and pour in ¼ cup of the batter. Quickly tilt the pan in all directions, coating the bottom with a thin, even film of batter. Return the pan to the heat and cook until the crepe bubbles, about 45 seconds. Turn the crepe and cook the other side for about 30 seconds.
6. Stack the crepes on a plate for filling.

MAKES ABOUT 16 CREPES

Calories	Total Protein	Soy Protein	Carbohydrate	Fat	Cholesterol	Fiber	Sodium
75	4.5 g	1 g	12 g	2 g	0 mg	2 g	70 mg

Information is for 1 crepe.

Variation: For a simple and sweet brunch treat, fold finished crepes into quarters, sprinkle them with confectioners' sugar, and spoon a dollop of strawberry jam on top.

Soy Crepes with Ratatouille

These Mediterranean-style crepes enclose a filling inspired by the traditional Provençal vegetable stew of eggplant, zucchini, tomatoes, and onions. Ratatouille is usually cooked for a long time, until the vegetables soften and meld, but I find the flavor fresher in this light sauté. The crumbled tofu adds soy protein, of course, and also enables this ratatouille to stand alone as a side dish or light lunch.

½ small eggplant

Salt

2 tablespoons olive oil

½ medium red onion, thinly sliced

1 small zucchini, sliced into matchsticks

1 medium yellow squash, sliced into matchsticks

1 small red bell pepper, sliced into matchsticks

3 garlic cloves, minced

6 ounces soft tofu, crumbled

12 Soy Crepes (page 90)

1½ cups Tomato Sauce (page 111)

6 ounces soy mozzarella cheese, shredded

Salt and pepper to taste

1. Slice the eggplant and place on a cookie sheet. Sprinkle with salt and set aside for half an hour. Blot the moisture from the eggplant and slice into thin matchsticks.

2. In a large skillet, heat the oil over high heat and sauté the eggplant, onion, zucchini, yellow squash, peppers, and garlic for 5 minutes. Add the tofu and mix until thoroughly heated.

3. Preheat the oven to 375°F. Place about 3 tablespoons of vegetable filling on each crepe and roll into a cylinder. Place the filled crepes in a 9 × 13-inch baking dish and spoon the tomato sauce over them. Sprinkle shredded cheese on top and bake for 12 to 15 minutes until cheese is melted. Serve hot.

SERVES 6

Calories	Total Protein	Soy Protein	Carbohydrate	Fat	Cholesterol	Fiber	Sodium
249	13 g	9 g	23 g	12 g	0 mg	4 g	287 mg

Information is for 2 crepes.

Woodland Wild Mushroom Crepes

This is a hearty mushroom ragout, rolled in a delicate pancake shell and topped with a warm soy cheese sauce. The savory filling, flecked with tofu, is so delicious that it can stand on its own, served with a slice of toasted Soy Herb Bread (page 104). Though wild mushrooms are a luxury, they lend this dish a rich, earthy flavor that ordinary mushrooms can't match. If dried mushrooms are hard to find, however, substitute fresh mushrooms of your choice.

1½ cups dried mushrooms (morels, shiitakes, or other packaged wild mushrooms)

2 tablespoons vegetable oil

1 small onion, finely chopped

2 celery stalks, chopped

½ cup diced tomato (about 1 medium tomato)

6 ounces soft tofu, crumbled

½ teaspoon dried tarragon

Salt and pepper to taste

2 cups cooked brown rice

12 Soy Crepes (page 90)

1½ cups Soy Mornay Sauce (page 76), room temperature

1. Soak the mushrooms in warm water for half an hour to reconstitute. Drain and chop coarsely.

2. In a large saucepan, heat the oil over medium-high heat. Sauté the onion and celery until soft, about 5 minutes.

3. Add the diced tomato, tofu, and mushrooms, sautéing about 5 minutes. Season with tarragon, salt, and pepper. The mixture will be rather dry.

4. Add the brown rice to the mushroom mixture and heat through, about 3 minutes.

5. Preheat the oven to 350°F. Fill each crepe with about 3 tablespoons of stuffing and roll into a cylinder.

6. Place the crepes in a shallow 9 × 13-inch baking pan and spoon the sauce over them. Bake for 15 minutes or until sauce is hot. Serve immediately.

SERVES 6

Calories	Total Protein	Soy Protein	Carbohydrate	Fat	Cholesterol	Fiber	Sodium
441	14 g	12 g	55 g	15 g	0 mg	4 g	488 mg

Information is for 2 crepes.

Blintzes

Blintzes, a delectable Eastern European dish of thin pancakes enclosing a sweet, rich, cream cheese filling, were always my favorite treats at family celebrations. I've created a healthful version, in which soy cream cheese takes the place of cholesterol-laden dairy cheese, providing 24 grams of soy protein per serving. No one I've served them to has ever noticed the difference.

24 ounces soy cream cheese, at room temperature

½ cup sugar

2 teaspoons vanilla extract

Zest of 2 small lemons, minced

12 Soy Crepes (page 90)

2 tablespoons soy margarine, melted (optional)

6 tablespoons strawberry preserves

1. Preheat the oven to 325°F. Combine the cream cheese, sugar, vanilla, and lemon zest in a medium bowl. Stir until smooth.
2. Fill each crepe with 3 tablespoons filling.
3. Roll the crepes up and brush with the melted soy margarine. Place them in a shallow 9 × 13-inch baking dish and heat for 15 minutes or until warm. Place 2 crepes on each plate, along with a tablespoon of preserves.

SERVES 6

Calories	Total Protein	Soy Protein	Carbohydrate	Fat	Cholesterol	Fiber	Sodium
480	30 g	24 g	28 g	38 g	5 mg	2 g	291 mg

Information is for 2 blintzes.

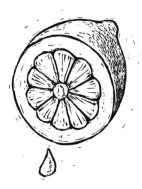

Soy Milk Biscuits

Slightly denser than regular biscuits, these are incredible served hot from the oven with strawberry jam or honey.

2 cups unbleached all-purpose flour

3 teaspoons baking powder

¾ teaspoon salt

6 tablespoons soy margarine, chilled

¾ cup soy milk

1. Preheat the oven to 425°F. Lightly grease a baking sheet or line it with parchment paper.

2. Sift the flour, baking powder, and salt together into a large mixing bowl and set aside.

3. Cut the margarine into the flour until the mixture resembles coarse crumbs. Stir in the soy milk and form the dough into a ball.

4. On a floured surface, roll the dough out about 2 inches thick. Cut into 2-inch rounds with a biscuit or cookie cutter.

5. Place the biscuits on the baking sheet and bake for 15 minutes, until slightly brown. Serve immediately.

MAKES 12 BISCUITS

Calories	Total Protein	Soy Protein	Carbohydrate	Fat	Cholesterol	Fiber	Sodium
132	2.5 g	0.5 g	16 g	6 g	0 mg	0.5 g	220 mg

Information is for 1 biscuit.

Variations: *Cheese Biscuits:* Add 2 ounces of grated soy cheddar to the dry ingredients. *Cinnamon Raisin Biscuits:* Add 1 ounce of raisins to the dry ingredients and sprinkle the biscuit tops with cinnamon sugar before baking. *Herbed Biscuits:* Add 2 teaspoons of any dried herb mixture to the dry ingredients.

Whole Wheat Banana Soy Muffins

Heaped in a basket on a brunch table, or offered to hungry children as a nutritious after-school snack, these muffins will disappear fast. With no eggs, they turn out moist, somewhat dense, and packed with banana flavor. For great taste and a little crunch, you can add up to ¼ cup of chopped walnuts.

>2 cups whole wheat pastry flour
>½ teaspoon salt
>1 tablespoon baking powder
>2 large, very ripe bananas
>⅓ cup vegetable oil
>¼ cup honey
>½ cup soy milk

1. Preheat the oven to 350°F. and grease a 12-cup muffin tin.
2. Combine the flour, salt, and baking powder in a large mixing bowl.
3. Puree the bananas in a food processor or blender and transfer to medium mixing bowl. Add the oil, honey, and soy milk and mix well.
4. Pour the banana mixture into the dry ingredients and stir just until moistened.
5. Pour the batter into the greased cups and bake for 30 minutes, until lightly brown and firm to the touch.

MAKES 12 MUFFINS

Calories	Total Protein	Soy Protein	Carbohydrate	Fat	Cholesterol	Fiber	Sodium
169	3.2 g	0.5 g	26 g	6 g	0 mg	3.5 g	174 mg

Information is for 1 muffin.

Carrot Soy Muffins

Moist and dense, this muffin may fool your sweet tooth into thinking it's getting a piece of carrot cake. These are delicious plain, or enriched with the addition of a ½ cup of golden raisins and a teaspoon of cinnamon. You can easily turn these into cupcakes by frosting them with soy cream cheese, whipped in a blender or food processor until fluffy.

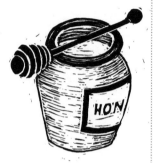

2 cups whole wheat pastry flour
½ teaspoon salt
2 teaspoons baking powder
1 cup finely grated carrots (about 2 medium)
⅓ cup vegetable oil
½ cup honey
½ cup soy milk

1. Preheat the oven to 350°F. and grease a 12-cup muffin tin.
2. Combine the flour, salt, and baking powder in a large mixing bowl. Stir in the grated carrots.
3. In a medium bowl, combine the oil, honey, and soy milk.
4. Pour the liquid mixture into the dry ingredients and mix just until moistened.
5. Fill the greased muffin cups and bake for 30 minutes, until lightly brown and firm to the touch.

MAKES 12 MUFFINS

Calories	Total Protein	Soy Protein	Carbohydrate	Fat	Cholesterol	Fiber	Sodium
152	3 g	1 g	21 g	6 g	0 mg	3.5 g	178 mg

Information is for 1 muffin.

Sweet Potato Soy Muffins

Try these with a cup of tea for an afternoon pick-me-up. The sweet potatoes make them so moist and sweet, you won't need to top them with butter or jelly.

2 cups whole wheat pastry flour

½ teaspoon salt

2 teaspoons baking powder

1 medium sweet potato, cooked, peeled, and mashed

⅓ cup vegetable oil

½ cup honey

½ cup soy milk

1. Preheat the oven to 350°F. and grease a 12-cup muffin tin.

2. Combine the flour, salt, and baking powder in a large mixing bowl.

3. In a medium bowl, combine the sweet potato, oil, honey, and soy milk, mixing thoroughly.

4. Pour the sweet potato mixture into the dry ingredients, and mix just until combined.

5. Fill the greased muffin cups and bake for 30 minutes, until lightly brown and firm to the touch.

MAKES 12 MUFFINS

Calories	Total Protein	Soy Protein	Carbohydrate	Fat	Cholesterol	Fiber	Sodium
168	3 g	0.5 g	25 g	6 g	0 mg	3.5 g	190 mg

Information is for 1 muffin.

Peanut Butter Muffins

Peanut butter muffins? Why not? Peanut butter cookies are yummy—and the nutty flavor is every bit as good in muffins. Plus, the combination of peanut butter and soy milk in these provides more protein than most muffins. These moist, rich goodies are delicious plain, or try them with—what else?—a little jelly. Hint: warming the peanut butter and honey slightly in a microwave oven makes them easier to mix.

> 2 cups whole wheat pastry flour
> ½ teaspoon salt
> 1 tablespoon baking powder
> ¼ cup creamy peanut butter
> ⅓ cup vegetable oil
> ¼ cup honey
> ½ cup soy milk

1. Preheat the oven to 350°F. Grease a 12-cup muffin tin.
2. In a large mixing bowl, combine the flour, salt, and baking powder.
3. In a medium mixing bowl, beat the peanut butter, oil, honey, and soy milk together until smooth. Add the dry ingredients and stir with a wooden spoon until just combined.
4. Pour the batter into the muffin cups and bake for 25 minutes, until lightly brown and firm to the touch.

MAKES 12 MUFFINS

Calories	Total Protein	Soy Protein	Carbohydrate	Fat	Cholesterol	Fiber	Sodium
178	4.6 g	0.5 g	21 g	9 g	0 mg	3.7 g	175 mg

Information is for 1 muffin.

Soy Cheese Corn Bread

This hearty, whole wheat corn bread means business. It's moist and protein-packed, thanks to the soy milk and zesty grated cheddar. Depending on your preference, you can make bread or muffins from this recipe. Either is the perfect complement to dishes like Soybean Chili (page 134) because the cornmeal in the bread and the soybeans in the chili combine to form a complete protein. Hint: a teaspoon of minced jalapeño pepper in the batter adds zip.

1¼ cups whole wheat flour

¾ cup yellow cornmeal

2 teaspoons baking powder

½ teaspoon salt

¼ cup sugar

1½ cups soy milk

2 tablespoons vegetable oil

6 ounces soy cheddar cheese, grated

1. Preheat the oven to 400°F. Grease an 8 × 8-inch square pan or a 12-cup muffin tin.

2. In a large mixing bowl, combine the flour, cornmeal, baking powder, salt, and sugar and set aside.

3. In a medium bowl, combine the soy milk and oil. Fold the flour mixture into the soy milk mixture, stirring until just moistened.

4. Add the cheese when thoroughly mixed.

5. Place in the greased pan or muffin tin and bake for 25 minutes, or until wooden pick inserted into the middle of the pan comes out clean.

MAKES 9 PIECES OF CORN BREAD OR 12 MUFFINS

Calories	Total Protein	Soy Protein	Carbohydrate	Fat	Cholesterol	Fiber	Sodium
164	5.6 g	3.5 g	19 g	7 g	0 mg	3 g	143 mg

Information is for 1 piece of corn bread or muffin.

Soy Date Walnut Loaf

Slather slices of this dark, sweet date loaf with soy cream cheese for a delectable treat with coffee, or serve with fruit salad for a fabulous lunch. Hint: to make even slices, refrigerate the loaf for an hour before cutting.

2 cups whole wheat pastry flour
1 tablespoon baking powder
½ teaspoon salt
⅓ cup vegetable oil
¼ cup honey
½ cup soy milk
½ cup chopped dates
½ cup chopped walnuts

1. Preheat the oven to 350°F. Grease a 9 × 5-inch loaf pan or line with parchment paper, letting the ends hang over the sides of the pan.
2. In a medium mixing bowl, combine the flour, baking powder, and salt.
3. In a large bowl, combine the oil, honey, and soy milk.
4. Add the flour mixture to the soy milk mixture, stirring just until moistened. Gently fold in the dates and walnuts.
5. Pour the batter into the prepared pan and bake for 40 minutes or until wooden pick inserted into the middle of the cake comes out clean.

MAKES 1 12-SLICE LOAF

Calories	Total Protein	Soy Protein	Carbohydrate	Fat	Cholesterol	Fiber	Sodium
199	4.4 g	5 g	26 g	9 g	0 mg	4 g	174 mg

Information is for 1 slice.

Soy Sour Cream Lemon Loaf

A soy version of all-American pound cake, this loaf has no eggs, butter, or cream but tastes remarkably similar. Have a slice with your morning coffee or as a snack. Or serve it warm as a simple dessert, with a scoop of Tofu Ice Cream (page 209) or frozen yogurt.

2 cups whole wheat flour
1 tablespoon baking powder
½ teaspoon salt
Zest of ½ lemon, grated
2 tablespoons egg replacer
½ cup water

¾ cup soy margarine, softened to
   room temperature
1 cup sugar
1 cup soy sour cream
1 teaspoon vanilla extract

1. Preheat the oven to 325°F. Grease a 9 × 5-inch loaf pan or line it with parchment paper, letting the ends hang over the sides of the pan.
2. In a large bowl, combine the flour, baking powder, salt, and lemon zest and mix well.
3. Beat the egg replacer and water with an electric mixer until thoroughly combined. Add the margarine and sugar, beating until fluffy and almost white in color. Add the sour cream and vanilla and continue to beat until all the ingredients are well combined.
4. Add the liquid mixture to the dry ingredients and mix until combined. Fill the loaf pan with the mixture. Bake for 1 hour, or until wooden pick inserted into the middle of the loaf comes out clean. Cool completely before removing parchment and serving.

MAKES 1 12-SLICE LOAF

Calories	Total Protein	Soy Protein	Carbohydrate	Fat	Cholesterol	Fiber	Sodium
322	3 g	1 g	24.5 g	14 g	0 mg	2 g	384 mg

Information is for 1 slice.

Soy Challah

Challah is a slightly sweet, traditional Jewish Sabbath bread normally made with and glazed with eggs. This version, braided like the original and topped with sesame or poppy seeds, is a delicious, cholesterol-free treat. Challah is versatile enough to be served at any meal, but I especially like it at brunch, toasted and spread with honey or jam.

1 cup lukewarm water

1 package fast-acting dry yeast

2 tablespoons sugar

⅓ cup soy milk, plus additional for brushing loaves

2 tablespoons vegetable oil

3 cups unbleached all-purpose flour, plus more for kneading

1 teaspoon salt

2 tablespoons sesame or poppy seeds

1. In a large mixing bowl, combine the water, yeast, and sugar, stirring until dissolved.

2. Add soy milk and oil, mixing thoroughly.

3. Gradually stir in the flour and salt. Using a large rubber spatula or wooden spoon, mix until combined.

4. Transfer the dough to a floured surface and knead for 3 to 4 minutes, or until dough is smooth and elastic. Sprinkle on a little more flour as needed to prevent stickiness.

5. Place the dough in a clean, lightly oiled bowl and cover with plastic wrap. Let rise in a warm place for 1½ hours, until doubled in bulk.

6. Preheat the oven to 350° F. Remove the risen dough to a floured board and with your hands, flatten it into a circle. Divide the dough into 6 equal parts.

7. Roll each part into a rope 1½ inches wide and 12 inches long. Using 3 ropes, form a braid, pressing the ends together neatly. Do the same with the remaining 3 ropes. Line a cookie sheet with parchment paper and place the loaves on it. Brush the loaves with soy milk and sprinkle with sesame or poppy seeds. Let the loaves rest for 10 minutes.

8. Bake for 35 to 40 minutes, until golden brown.

Calories	Total Protein	Soy Protein	Carbohydrate	Fat	Cholesterol	Fiber	Sodium
162	4.7 g	1 g	28 g	3 g	0 mg	1 g	181 mg

Information is for 1 slice.

Variations: *Whole Wheat Challah:* Substitute 3 cups of whole wheat flour for all-purpose flour. *Raisin Challah:* Knead ½ cup of raisins into the dough in step 6.

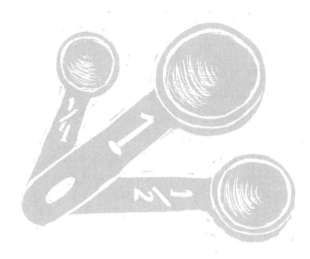

Soy Herb Bread

Nothing could be more satisfying than a warm slice of this fragrant bread alongside a bowl of steaming soup . . . or laden with melted soy cheddar or wrapped around slices of a juicy, garden tomato. The combination of thyme, oregano, and rosemary produces a Provençal flavor, but you can experiment with herbs of your choice, such as dill or basil. Yeast breads made with soy products have the same texture as ordinary breads; you'll never know you sneaked in some soy goodness.

1 cup lukewarm water	1 teaspoon salt
1 package fast-acting dry yeast	2 tablespoons dried thyme
2 tablespoons sugar	2 tablespoons dried oregano
⅓ cup soy milk	2 tablespoons dried rosemary
2 tablespoons vegetable oil	
3 cups unbleached all-purpose flour, plus more for kneading	

1. In a large mixing bowl, combine the water, yeast, and sugar. Stir until dissolved.

2. Add the soy milk and oil, mixing thoroughly.

3. Gradually stir in the flour and salt, mixing with a wooden spoon until combined.

4. Transfer the dough to a floured surface and sprinkle on the herbs. Knead for 3 to 4 minutes, or until the dough is smooth and elastic.

5. Place the dough in a clean, lightly oiled bowl and cover with plastic wrap. Let rise in a warm place for 1½ hours, until doubled in bulk.

6. Divide the dough in half and form each half into a ball.

7. Place the loaves on a greased cookie sheet and bake at 350°F. for 35 to 40 minutes, until golden brown.

MAKES 2 6-SLICE LOAVES

Calories	Total Protein	Soy Protein	Carbohydrate	Fat	Cholesterol	Fiber	Sodium
162	4.7 g	1 g	28 g	3 g	0 mg	1 g	181 mg

Information is for 1 slice.

Soy Olive Bread

Imported olives add flavor to this fragrant bread, which brings out the best in Mediterranean-style dishes such as Soybean Minestrone (page 127) or Fusilli with Soy Pesto (page 169). This makes two loaves; the extra loaf can be frozen, wrapped tightly, for future use.

1 cup lukewarm water

1 package fast-acting dry yeast

2 tablespoons sugar

⅓ cup soy milk

2 tablespoons vegetable oil

3 cups unbleached all-purpose
  flour, plus more for kneading

1 teaspoon salt

½ cup pitted and thinly sliced
  Kalamata olives

1. Pour the water into a large mixing bowl and add the yeast and sugar. Stir until dissolved.

2. Add the soy milk and oil, mixing thoroughly. Using a wooden spoon, gradually stir in the flour and salt. Add the olives.

3. Transfer the dough to a floured board and knead for 3 to 4 minutes, until it is smooth and elastic.

4. Place the dough in a clean, lightly oiled bowl, cover with plastic wrap, and let rise in a warm place for 1½ hours, until doubled in bulk.

5. Preheat the oven to 350°F. Divide the dough in half and form each half into a round loaf.

6. Put the loaves on a greased cookie sheet and bake at 350°F. for 35 to 40 minutes, until golden brown.

MAKES 2 6-SLICE LOAVES

Calories	Total Protein	Soy Protein	Carbohydrate	Fat	Cholesterol	Fiber	Sodium
162	4.7 g	1 g	28 g	3 g	0 mg	1 g	181 mg

Information is for 1 slice.

Soy Whole Wheat Bread

Aha! Here is the perfect sandwich bread. After you take it out of the oven, inhale its heavenly aroma, tap its golden crust, and slice off "just a few slices" to sample, there's not likely to be enough left to make sandwiches from!

4 cups whole wheat flour, plus more for kneading
½ cup soy flour
1 teaspoon salt
1¾ cups soy milk
⅓ cup molasses
2 tablespoons vegetable oil
2 packages fast-acting dry yeast

1. Combine the flours and salt in a medium bowl and set aside.
2. In a small saucepan, over low heat, warm the soy milk, molasses, and oil until slightly warm (about 110°F.), stirring constantly.
3. Pour the milk mixture into a large mixing bowl. Add the yeast and mix thoroughly. Set aside for 5 minutes, until yeast mixture is foamy.
4. Using a wooden spoon, gradually stir in the flour mixture a little at a time until a soft dough is formed. Transfer the dough to a lightly floured surface and knead until it is smooth and elastic, about 3 to 4 minutes.
5. Shape the dough into a ball and place it in a lightly oiled bowl. Cover and let rise in a warm place for about 1½ hours, until doubled in bulk.
6. Preheat the oven to 375°F. Grease a 9×5-inch loaf pan. Remove the dough from the bowl and flatten it out with your hands. Shape dough into a loaf and place it in the pan.
7. Bake for 35 to 40 minutes, until golden brown.

MAKES 1 12-SLICE LOAF

Calories	Total Protein	Soy Protein	Carbohydrate	Fat	Cholesterol	Fiber	Sodium
190	7 g	1 g	34 g	4 g	0 mg	6 g	192 mg

Information is for 1 slice.

Pumpernickel Bread

What gives hearty pumpernickel bread its gorgeous mahogany color? The secret ingredients are strong coffee and cocoa powder, though you'd never guess it from the taste. Slightly sweet from the molasses and fragrant from the traditional caraway seeds, this German-style bread is fabulous for sandwiches or for breakfast, slathered with soy cream cheese. For a variation, try adding ½ cup dark raisins when forming loaves for baking.

2 cups lukewarm water

2 packages fast-acting dry yeast

¼ cup dark molasses

½ cup soy milk

¼ cup vegetable oil

2 tablespoons strong black coffee

1 tablespoon unsweetened cocoa powder

3 cups rye flour

4 cups unbleached all-purpose flour

2 teaspoons salt

1½ tablespoons caraway seeds

1. Pour the water into a large mixing bowl and add the yeast and molasses. Stir until dissolved. Add the soy milk, oil, and coffee, mixing thoroughly.

2. Gradually stir in the cocoa powder, rye flour, and 3 cups of all-purpose flour and salt. Mix until combined, using a stout wooden spoon, as the dough will be stiff. Add some more flour as needed so dough isn't sticky.

3. Transfer the dough to a floured surface, sprinkle the caraway seeds, and knead for 3 to 4 minutes. Dust the dough with the remaining flour as necessary and continue kneading until it is smooth and elastic.

4. Place the dough in a clean, lightly oiled bowl, cover with plastic wrap, and let rise in a warm place for 1½ hours, until doubled in bulk.

5. Preheat the oven to 350°F. Divide the dough in half and form each half into a ball.

6. Put the loaves on a greased cookie sheet and bake for 35 to 40 minutes, until top of the loaves brown.

MAKES 2 12-SLICE LOAVES

Calories	Total Protein	Soy Protein	Carbohydrate	Fat	Cholesterol	Fiber	Sodium
164	5 g	0.25 g	28.5 g	3 g	0 mg	1 g	183 mg

Information is for 1 slice.

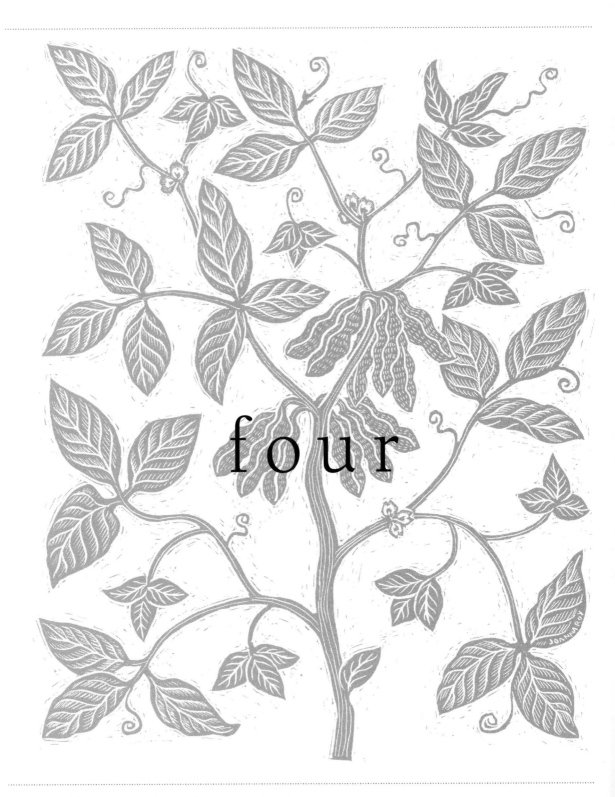

four

pizza and sandwiches

What's more universally beloved than pizza, with its hot, crisp crust covered with tomato sauce and dripping melted cheese? Pizza is always a hit-the-spot snack or a satisfying meal. Unfortunately, however, it can also be very high in fat and cholesterol. But in these recipes, soy transforms pizza from everyone's favorite "fun" food to serious nutrition.

Start with a homemade crust that contains soy flour. Top it with fresh tomato sauce and shredded soy mozzarella cheese. Add crumbled soy sausage and onions, or soy pepperoni and mushrooms, and the final product provides a substantial amount of health-giving soy protein with only one quarter of the fat of regular pizza. If you're short on time, you'll enjoy my no-fuss Soy Sausage Tortilla Pizza just as much. It uses ready-made foods products in place of the homemade crust.

You will also love pizza's first cousin, focaccia. Focaccia is a raised bread, thicker than a pizza crust, that is served plain or lightly topped with onions, herbs, meats, or cheese. Depending on its topping, it can be a meal in itself or a complement to other dishes. Here, soy flour enhances the dough and soy cheese and sausage add substance.

With soy foods, you can grab a quick sandwich—grilled soy cheddar on Soy Whole Wheat Bread (page 106), for example—and still get plenty of good nutrition. Who needs hamburgers when you've got Tofu Spinach Burgers, with 4.5 grams of soy protein or Soy Sloppy Joes, with an incredible 29 grams of soy protein?

Surprise! Soy has turned pizza and burgers into health food.

Pizza Variations

Use your imagination to create limitless pizza variations. For example, add a finely minced garlic clove and a little oregano, basil, or rosemary to the dough, to give flavor to the crust.

Before sprinkling on the soy mozzarella, top the pizza with:

• Soy pepperoni and sliced mushrooms

• Grilled strips of eggplant, red and green peppers, and thin rings of red onion

• Soy ham and chunks of pineapple

• Crumbled cooked soy sausage, black olives, minced garlic, and red pepper flakes

Soy Cheese Pizza

This pizza looks and tastes so much like the real thing that you won't know the difference. I've replaced the usual mozzarella cheese with soy mozzarella, which melts beautifully at high temperatures. A little soy flour adds nutritional punch to the crust without affecting the taste or texture. The simple homemade tomato sauce has a fresh lively flavor. Hint: baking this on a preheated pizza stone will produce a crisper crust.

1 cup warm water

1 package fast-acting yeast

2 tablespoons olive oil

2 cups unbleached all-purpose flour, plus more for kneading

½ cup soy flour

¾ teaspoon salt

Cornmeal, for dusting

2 cups Tomato Sauce (page 111)

1 tablespoon Italian seasoning

12 ounces soy mozzarella cheese, shredded

1. In a small bowl, combine the warm water, yeast, and olive oil.

2. In a large bowl, combine the flours and salt.

3. Add the yeast mixture to the dry ingredients and stir with a rubber spatula until a soft dough forms.

4. Transfer the dough to a floured surface, and knead until the dough is smooth and elastic, about 5 minutes.

5. Cover with plastic wrap and let sit for 10 minutes.

6. Preheat the oven to 450°F. Lightly oil a 14-inch pizza pan, sprinkle with cornmeal, and shape dough to fit the pan.

7. Top the pizza dough with the tomato sauce, Italian seasoning, and soy cheese.

8. Bake for 10 minutes, or until crust is crisp and cheese is bubbly.

SERVES 6

Calories	Total Protein	Soy Protein	Carbohydrate	Fat	Cholesterol	Fiber	Sodium
279	10 g	3 g	42 g	7 g	0 mg	3.7 g	398 mg

Information is 1 slice.

Soy Sausage Tortilla Pizzas

These tasty snack pizzas, studded with meaty soy sausage and blanketed with bubbling cheese, are real time-savers. They start out with ready-made, whole wheat tortillas rather than a pizza crust, so you can whip them up in about 15 minutes.

1 tablespoon vegetable oil

6 ounces soy sausage

1½ teaspoons Italian seasoning

1½ teaspoons minced garlic

½ cup Tomato Sauce (see sidebar)

6 whole wheat tortillas

8 ounces soy mozzarella cheese, shredded

1. In a medium saucepan, heat the oil over medium-high heat and cook the sausage until it browns, breaking up into small chunks and stirring to prevent sticking. Add the Italian seasoning, garlic, and tomato sauce and heat thoroughly.

2. Preheat the broiler.

3 Put an even amount of the sausage mixture on each whole wheat tortilla, and top with the soy mozzarella.

4. Broil for 5 minutes, or until slightly browned. Serve hot.

SERVES 6

Calories	Total Protein	Soy Protein	Carbohydrate	Fat	Cholesterol	Fiber	Sodium
246	15 g	13 g	23 g	10 g	0 mg	1 g	408 mg

Information is for 1 tortilla.

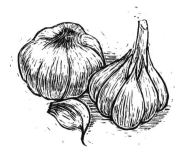

Tomato Sauce

2 tablespoons olive oil

1 large onion, chopped

3 garlic cloves, minced

1 medium carrot, chopped

1 celery stalk, chopped

1 tablespoon Italian seasoning

2 teaspoons dried rosemary

2 teaspoons dried oregano

Salt and pepper to taste

1 28-ounce can tomatoes (or 1½ pounds fresh), coarsely chopped

1. Heat the oil in large saucepan over medium-high heat and sauté the onion until translucent, about 5 minutes. Add the garlic, carrot, and celery and sauté for 3 more minutes.

2. Stir in the Italian seasoning, rosemary, oregano, and salt and pepper, cooking 2 to 3 minutes more.

3. Add the tomatoes, reduce the heat to low, cover, and simmer for 1 hour. Sauce may be left chunky or pureed in a food processor or blender.

MAKES 6 CUPS

Calories: 64, Total Protein: 2 g,	
Soy Protein: 0 g,	
Carbohydrate: 10 g, Fat: 2.5 g,	
Cholesterol: 0 mg, Fiber: 3 g,	
Sodium: 196 mg	

Information is per serving.

Onion Soy Parmesan Focaccia

Focaccia is a versatile Italian yeast bread, sort of like a very airy, high pizza crust flavored with herbs and olive oil. Like pizza, it can be topped with any number of ingredients. You can really go crazy with toppings, if you like: try adding roasted red peppers and garlic, or soy mozzarella and pesto, for example. I like to serve this healthful bread as a snack or appetizer, accompanied by a bowl of warm tomato sauce for dipping. It will freeze well, tightly wrapped, up to three months.

1 cup warm water

1 cup soy milk

1 package active dry yeast

2 tablespoons sugar

3 cups unbleached all-purpose
  flour, plus more for kneading

½ cup soy flour

1 teaspoon salt

½ teaspoon white pepper

2 teaspoons dried basil

Cornmeal, for dusting

1 tablespoon olive oil

½ small onion, finely chopped

¼ cup soy parmesan cheese

1. Combine the water, soy milk, yeast, and sugar in a large bowl and stir until yeast is dissolved and foamy, about 5 minutes.

2. In a large bowl, combine the flours, salt, pepper, and basil, and gradually add the yeast liquid, mixing thoroughly with a rubber spatula until a soft dough forms.

3. Transfer the dough to a floured surface and knead for 8 to 10 minutes, or until dough is no longer sticky.

4. Form dough into a ball and place in a slightly oiled bowl. Cover and let rise until doubled, about 1 hour.

5. Preheat the oven to 400°F. Line a 11 × 17-inch baking sheet with parchment paper and sprinkle with cornmeal.

6. Heat the olive oil over medium-high heat and sauté the onion until translucent, about 5 minutes. Set aside to cool.

7. Flatten the dough on a floured surface and roll out into a rectangle to fit on the baking sheet, about 10×15 inches. Sprinkle the top with sautéed onion and the soy parmesan. Bake for 20 minutes, until golden brown. Cut into squares and serve hot.

MAKES 8 LARGE PIECES OR 32 HORS D'OEUVRES

Calories	Total Protein	Soy Protein	Carbohydrate	Fat	Cholesterol	Fiber	Sodium
220	7 g	1 g	40 g	3 g	0 mg	2 g	360 mg

Information is for 1 large piece.

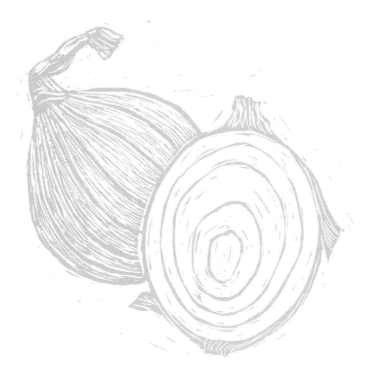

Soy Sausage Stuffed Focaccia

Focaccia dough is folded over a rich filling of soy sausage and mozzarella, making a delectable surprise when you cut it into squares. Serve this as a hearty appetizer or, cut into larger pieces, as the basis for a meal, accompanied by a green salad with Creamy Herb Dressing (page 72).

> 1 recipe focaccia dough (page 112)
> 2 tablespoons olive oil
> ½ small onion, finely chopped
> 1 14-ounce package soy sausage
> 4 ounces soy mozzarella cheese, shredded

1. Prepare the focaccia according to the recipe through step 5.
2. Heat the oil in a saucepan over medium-high heat and sauté the onion until it is translucent, about 5 minutes. Set aside. In the same pan, brown the sausage, breaking it up into small pieces. Set aside.
3. Flatten the dough on a floured surface and roll out to a rectangle about 10 × 15 inches. With the short side of the dough facing you, sprinkle the onion on the lower half. Follow the onion with the crumbled sausage and the soy mozzarella. Leave a 1-inch border at the edges.
4. Fold the plain half of the dough over the topping and pinch the edges together. Bake for 25 minutes or until golden brown. Cut into squares and serve hot.

SERVES 8

Calories	Total Protein	Soy Protein	Carbohydrate	Fat	Cholesterol	Fiber	Sodium
325	19 g	13 g	49 g	5.5g	0 mg	4 g	525 mg

Information is for 1 piece.

Almond Soy-Cheese Burger

A nutty vegetarian version of the all-American hamburger, this patty gets its robust flavor from ground nuts, seeds, and soy cheese spiked with a little chili powder. Try this on a whole wheat bun, dripping with fresh salsa.

½ cup almonds

½ cup soy nuts

½ cup sunflower seeds

4 ounces soy cheddar cheese, shredded

1 cup whole wheat bread crumbs

3 teaspoons ground cumin

3 teaspoons chili powder

¾ tablespoon dried oregano

2 tablespoons chopped parsley

1 scallion, sliced, green and white parts

¼ teaspoon black pepper

¾ cup soy milk

6 whole wheat buns

Lettuce, tomato, mustard, ketchup, salsa, or condiments of your choice, for garnish

1. Place the almonds, soy nuts, sunflower seeds, soy cheddar, and bread crumbs in a blender container. Blend on medium speed until the mixture resembles coarse meal.

2. Transfer to a large mixing bowl and add the cumin, chili powder, oregano, parsley, scallion, and pepper, mixing well. Add the soy milk, using a rubber spatula to combine the ingredients thoroughly. The mixture should resemble uncooked meat loaf.

3. Preheat the broiler. Form the mixture into 6 individual patties and broil for 3 minutes on each side, until firm and brown. Serve the patties on whole wheat buns, garnished to taste.

SERVES 6

Calories	Total Protein	Soy Protein	Carbohydrate	Fat	Cholesterol	Fiber	Sodium
318	16 g	8 g	38 g	14 g	0 mg	6.5 g	265 mg

Information is for 1 burger, including bun and garnishes.

Sandwich Suggestions

In a hurry for lunch? With soy foods, you can whip up great sandwiches that don't sacrifice good nutrition and good taste for ease of preparation. For example:

• Grill slices of soy cheddar cheese between slices of Soy Whole Wheat Bread (page 106). For a spicy change of pace, use soy jalapeño jack cheese.

• Spread a layer of soy cream cheese between two slices of Soy Date Walnut Loaf (page 100).

• Try Soy Almond Spread (page 49) and jelly on Soy Whole Wheat Bread (page 106).

• Spread Soy herb and garlic cream cheese on sliced Soy Olive Bread (page 105), add roasted red peppers and arugula, and top with another slice of bread.

• Layer crisp soy bacon, lettuce, and tomato, along with Tofu Mayonnaise (page 59), on Soy Whole Wheat Bread (page 106).

• Spread two slices of Soy Herb Bread (page 104) with Tofu Mayonnaise (page 59), layer avocado, slices of soy jack cheese and fresh tomato, and alfalfa sprouts.

Tofu Spinach Burgers

Protein-packed tofu takes the place of ground beef in this vegetarian burger. Tofu, spinach, garlic, onions, herbs, and spices, bound together with cracker meal, and topped with melted cheddar cheese, make these patties delicious served open-faced or tucked into a whole wheat bun. Because they contain no meat, fat, or eggs to firm them, the patties, like any vegetable burger, may fall apart easily. To help prevent this, use a food processor to mix the ingredients rapidly and thoroughly.

1 10-ounce package frozen spinach (chopped, not whole leaf), thawed

12 ounces low-fat firm tofu, crumbled

1½ cups crushed crackers (water crackers, matzoh, or soda crackers)

¼ medium onion, chopped

2 scallions, sliced, green and white parts

4 garlic cloves, minced

1 tablespoon dried tarragon

1 teaspoon dried sage

1 teaspoon dried thyme

½ teaspoon salt

½ teaspoon pepper

3 ounces soy cheddar cheese, shredded (optional)

1. Squeeze excess moisture from the spinach. Preheat the broiler.

2. In a food processor bowl, combine all the ingredients except the cheese and process just until the mixture reaches a uniform consistency and holds together.

3. Form into 6 patties and broil for 5 minutes on each side, until slightly brown. Top with the cheese during the last minute, if desired. Serve immediately, plain or on a bun.

SERVES 6

Calories	Total Protein	Soy Protein	Carbohydrate	Fat	Cholesterol	Fiber	Sodium
141	9 g	4.5 g	23 g	3 g	0 mg	8 g	229 mg

Information is for 1 burger, including bun.

Soy Sloppy Joes

Every bit as messy and great-tasting as the original beef version, these hearty sandwiches use soy sausage and take just minutes to prepare. They are a big hit with kids.

2 tablespoons vegetable oil

3 14-ounce packages soy sausage

1 medium onion, chopped

1 cup ketchup

2 cups tomato juice

2 tablespoons brown mustard

1 teaspoon salt

¼ teaspoon black pepper

6 whole-grain burger buns, split

1. In a large saucepan, heat the oil over medium heat and sauté the sausage and onion, stirring frequently to prevent sticking, until onion is translucent, about 5 minutes.

2. Add the ketchup, tomato juice, mustard, salt, and pepper, and simmer for 20 minutes, stirring frequently.

3. Smother each bun half with ½ cup of sausage mixture, replace bun top, and serve. (This mixture can be made ahead and frozen.)

SERVES 6

Calories	Total Protein	Soy Protein	Carbohydrate	Fat	Cholesterol	Fiber	Sodium
444	37 g	32 g	58 g	7 g	0 mg	5.5 g	1778 mg

Information is for 1 sloppy joe.

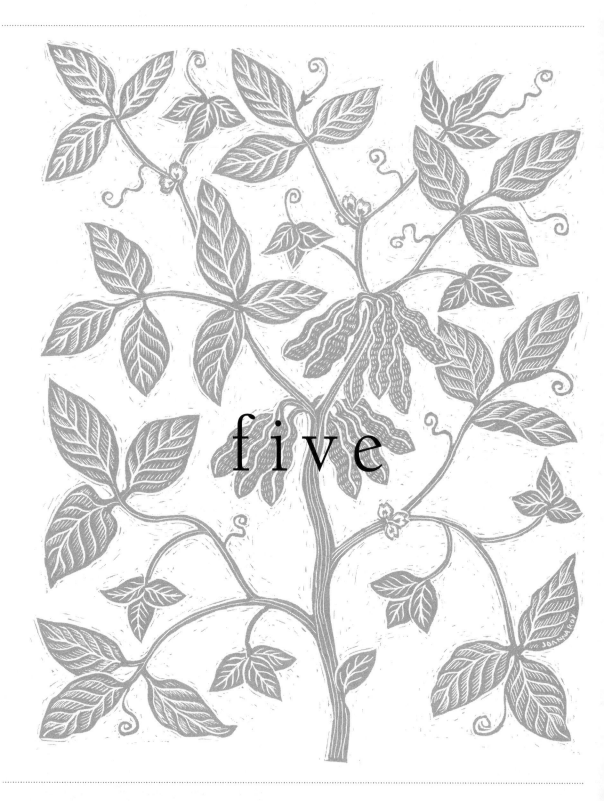

five

soups and stews

Nothing is more satisfying than making homemade soup—selecting and preparing the ingredients, then inhaling the aromas as the pot simmers on the stove. Unless, of course, you also happen to love *eating* homemade soup. What could be more perfect than a bowl of creamy tomato soup or spicy chili on a cold winter day? Well, possibly a refreshing cup of chilled cucumber soup on a sweltering August afternoon.

Soups and stews are a delicious disguise for balanced, nutritious meals. A friend of mine who has a whole family of picky eaters serves them split pea soup or minestrone all the time, and her children don't even notice that they are "eating their vegetables." For the same reason, soups and stews are ideal ways to introduce soy products to newcomers. A traditional soup such as vichyssoise, for example, tastes no different when made with soy milk instead of dairy milk. But it packs an enormously increased nutritional wallop. The soup recipes in this chapter use many different soy products in a number of ways. Cream of Asparagus is a silky puree made with soy milk; Soy Sausage Potato Chowder is made even heartier with tofu; Black Bean Chili with Tempeh is a chunky stew made with tempeh; and Soybean Minestrone and Soybean Chili feature whole soybeans.

Soups are a staple in my cooking, and I always make them in quantities large enough to freeze for those days when I'm just too busy to cook anything from scratch. Then I simply thaw an individual portion, make a salad, and serve with a few slices of crusty bread. All the soups in this chapter freeze well. Life just got a little easier!

Vegetable Stock

1 tablespoon vegetable oil
1 large onion, chopped
2 medium leeks, chopped, white part only
3 large carrots, chopped
3 celery stalks, chopped
4 garlic cloves, minced
8 cups water
1 teaspoon black peppercorns, slightly crushed
¼ cup chopped parsley
4 bay leaves, crushed

1. Heat the oil over medium-high heat in a large pot and sauté the onion, leeks, carrots, and celery until tender, about 8 minutes. Add the garlic and sauté a few minutes more.
2. Add the water, peppercorns, parsley, and bay leaves and bring to a boil. Reduce the heat and simmer, covered, for 2 hours, or, for more concentrated flavor, 4 hours.
3. Strain the stock, cool, and refrigerate or freeze.

MAKES 8 CUPS

Calories: 58, Total Protein: 1 g,
Soy Protein: 0 g, Carbohydrate: 10 g,
Fat: 2 g, Cholesterol: 0 mg, Fiber: 3 g,
Sodium: 37 mg
Information is for 1 cup.

Tofu Basil Soup

This delicious vegetable soup, studded with cubes of creamy tofu, gets its zingy Mediterranean flavor from fresh herbs, especially basil. If you try to substitute dried herbs, you may find the results disappointing. Luckily, fresh herbs are readily available in the produce sections of most markets. This soup starts out with vegetable stock. An easy recipe for fresh and flavorful homemade stock follows, because it comes in handy in so many recipes, it's a great idea to keep several quarts on hand in the freezer.

1 tablespoon olive oil
2 large carrots, chopped
2 celery stalks, chopped
½ small onion, chopped
1 medium leek, chopped
2 garlic cloves, minced
1 recipe Vegetable Stock (see sidebar)

2 tablespoons minced fresh oregano
1 sprig of fresh thyme
1 pound firm tofu, cubed
1 small bunch fresh basil, stems removed (12 to 16 leaves)
Salt and pepper to taste

1. Heat the oil in a large saucepan over medium heat and sauté the carrots, celery, onion, leek, and garlic until onion is translucent, about 5 minutes.
2. Add the stock, oregano, thyme, and tofu. Reduce the heat to low and simmer for 40 minutes.
3. Add the basil and simmer for another 10 minutes. Add salt and pepper and serve hot.

SERVES 6

Calories	Total Protein	Soy Protein	Carbohydrate	Fat	Cholesterol	Fiber	Sodium
65	6 g	6 g	2.6 g	4 g	0 mg	0 g	8 mg

Information is for a 1⅓-cup serving.

Miso Soup

A variation on the delicate soup served in Japanese restaurants, this gets its rich flavor from miso, a paste of fermented soybeans. Cubes of tofu and rounds of scallion fleck the deliciously simple broth. Serve this with Crispy Tofu with Plum and Ginger Sauce (page 35) or Tempeh Pepper "Steak" (page 149).

8 cups Vegetable Stock (page 120)

8 ounces yellow miso (available in health food stores and
   some large grocery stores)

4 ounces low-fat firm tofu, cut into small cubes

3 scallions, sliced, green and white parts

1. Bring the stock to a boil and reduce the heat to a simmer.
2. Add the miso and stir until heated through.
3. Pour into individual bowls. Divide the tofu cubes and sliced scallions among the bowls and serve at once.

SERVES 6

Calories	Total Protein	Soy Protein	Carbohydrate	Fat	Cholesterol	Fiber	Sodium
164	7 g	7 g	24 g	5 g	0 mg	6 g	1429 mg

Information is for a 1⅓-cup serving.

Chilled Cucumber Soup

No combination of flavors could be more refreshing in a summer soup than cucumbers, dill, and mint. Serve this soup the day it is made.

3 large cucumbers, peeled, seeded,
   and chopped

2 garlic cloves

4 fresh mint leaves

2 sprigs of dill

1 tablespoon honey

1 pound firm tofu

1 cup soy milk

1 teaspoon salt

3 scallions, sliced thinly, green and
   white parts

1. In a food processor or blender, puree the cucumbers, garlic, mint, and dill. Add the honey, tofu, and soy milk and blend until smooth.
2. Season with salt and chill for 1 hour. Garnish with sliced scallions.

SERVES 6

Calories	Total Protein	Soy Protein	Carbohydrate	Fat	Cholesterol	Fiber	Sodium
103	8 g	8 g	10 g	4.5 g	0 mg	2.5 g	369 mg

Information is for a 1-cup serving.

In soup recipes that call for tofu, such as Soy Hot and Sour Soup and Soy Sausage Potato Chowder, a useful trick to help the cubes hold their shape when simmering for long periods of time is to first freeze the cubed tofu overnight. The tofu will have a firmer, chewier consistency and will hold its shape a little better. To freeze, wrap the tofu tightly in plastic film or freezer bags. It will change color from white to light tan, but this will not affect the nutritional value. Thaw in the refrigerator overnight before using.

Soy Hot and Sour Soup

You'll think you've ordered in from your favorite Chinese restaurant when you taste this classic Mandarin-style soup. Chunks of tofu and soy ham, instead of the usual pork, float in a thick broth flavored by tangy vinegar and hot sauce. The only thing missing is the fortune cookie.

2 tablespoons cornstarch
¼ cup water
5 cups Vegetable Stock (page 120)
1 6-ounce can straw mushrooms, including juices
1 8-ounce can bamboo shoots, including juices
8 ounces extra-firm tofu, cubed
6 ounces soy ham, sliced
1 tablespoon soy sauce

1 teaspoon salt
2 tablespoons apple cider vinegar
¼ teaspoon white pepper
1 tablespoon sherry
½ teaspoon hot chili sauce (available in Asian or international section of supermarket, or use ordinary hot sauce)
Chopped cilantro, for garnish

1. In a small bowl, combine the cornstarch and water. Mix well.

2. Bring the stock to a boil in a large saucepan. Add the mushrooms and bamboo shoots, including their juices, and lower the heat to a simmer. Cook for 10 minutes.

3. Add the tofu, soy ham, soy sauce, salt, vinegar, pepper, sherry, and hot sauce, stirring well. Thoroughly mix in the cornstarch paste and cook over medium heat for 3 minutes, until slightly thickened.

4. Garnish with cilantro and serve immediately.

SERVES 6

Calories	Total Protein	Soy Protein	Carbohydrate	Fat	Cholesterol	Fiber	Sodium
143	12.2 g	10 g	17 g	3.5 g	0 mg	5.2 g	957 mg

Information is for a 1⅓-cup serving.

Carrot Ginger Soy Soup

This is a rich and creamy soup; the zip of ginger beautifully balances the sweetness of the carrots. I like to serve it at Thanksgiving because of its wonderful autumnal color, but it also makes a great summer lunch when served chilled, with Bombay Tempeh and Lentils (page 67).

1 tablespoon olive oil
6 medium carrots, chopped
2 medium onions, chopped
8 garlic cloves, chopped
4 cups Vegetable Stock (page 120)
2 cups low-fat soy milk
1 teaspoon salt
½ teaspoon white pepper
2 tablespoons ground ginger
½ cup soy sour cream, for garnish

1. Heat the oil in a large saucepan over medium-high heat and sauté the carrots and onions until the onions are translucent, about 5 minutes.

2. Add the garlic and continue to sauté until the carrots are softened, about 5 more minutes. Add small amounts of stock if the mixture gets too dry.

3. Add the stock, soy milk, salt, white pepper, and ginger. Reduce the heat to low and simmer for 20 more minutes.

4. Puree the soup in a blender and puree. Serve hot or cold, garnished with a dollop of soy sour cream.

SERVES 6

Calories	Total Protein	Soy Protein	Carbohydrate	Fat	Cholesterol	Fiber	Sodium
114	4 g	4 g	1 g	6 g	0 mg	3 g	294 mg

Information is for a 1⅓-cup serving, not including sour cream.

Cream of Asparagus Soup

Cream soups—those rich concoctions that so many people have given up for health reasons—become healthful choices when made with soy milk. I love this velvety pureed soup, with its delicate flavor and rich texture. And it's surprisingly easy to make!

¾ pound asparagus
1 tablespoon vegetable oil
1 small onion, finely chopped
¼ cup unbleached all-purpose flour
5 cups Vegetable Stock (page 120)
¾ cup soy milk
Salt and white pepper to taste

1. Remove and discard the tough stem parts of the asparagus. In a steamer basket set over boiling water, steam the asparagus for 2 minutes just to soften. Chop coarsely.
2. Heat the oil in a large, heavy saucepan over moderate heat. Add the onion and asparagus, and sauté for 3 minutes, without letting the onion brown.
3. Add the flour and cook, stirring, for 1 minute.
4. Gradually add the stock, continuing to stir until soup thickens, about 5 minutes.
5. Reduce the heat, add the soy milk, and simmer until the vegetables are tender, about 5 minutes. Puree the soup in a food processor or blender until smooth. Check for seasoning, adding salt and white pepper. Return to heat briefly if necessary; serve hot.

SERVES 6

Calories	Total Protein	Soy Protein	Carbohydrate	Fat	Cholesterol	Fiber	Sodium
107	3 g	1 g	8 g	2.5 g	0 mg	1.5 g	6 mg

Information is for a 1⅓-cup serving.

Cream of Tomato Soup

I wish I'd grown up on this luscious soup, instead of the one my family poured straight out of a can. This soy version is a lot more flavorful and nutritious than the original, and it tastes every bit as good with a grilled cheese sandwich.

1 tablespoon vegetable oil

1 medium onion, chopped

1 large carrot, chopped

1 celery stalk, chopped

2 garlic cloves, minced

6 ripe medium tomatoes, chopped

6 crushed black peppercorns

1 bay leaf

4 cups Vegetable Stock (page 120)

Salt to taste

2 cups soy milk

Parsley sprigs, for garnish

1. Heat the oil in a large pot over medium-high heat and sauté the onion, carrot, and celery until the onion starts to brown, about 8 minutes.

2. Add the garlic and sauté for 1 more minute. Lower the heat and add the tomatoes, peppercorns, and bay leaf, stirring well.

3. Add the stock and salt, and let the soup simmer for 35 minutes.

4. Remove from heat and allow to cool slightly. Remove bay leaf. Puree the soup in a food processor or blender until it is smooth. Pour the soup back into the pot through a fine-mesh strainer to remove any remaining solids and return to low heat. Stir in the soy milk and heat thoroughly. Serve immediately, garnished with parsley.

SERVES 6

Calories	Total Protein	Soy Protein	Carbohydrate	Fat	Cholesterol	Fiber	Sodium
64	3.5 g	3.5 g	9 g	2 g	0 mg	3 g	31 mg

Information is for a 1⅓-cup serving.

Soy Split Pea Soup

This soup cooks up thick and hearty. The yellow and green split peas add color contrast; the soy milk provides a creamy, nourishing base. For a spicy variation, add a tablespoon of either curry powder or chili powder as the soup simmers.

1 cup yellow split peas	3 garlic cloves, minced
1 cup green split peas	4 crushed black peppercorns
1 tablespoon vegetable oil	1 bay leaf
½ medium onion, chopped	6 cups Vegetable Stock (page 120)
2 large carrots, chopped	2 cups soy milk
2 celery stalks, chopped	Salt to taste
3 strips soy bacon, chopped (optional)	

1. Soak the yellow and green split peas together in about 6 cups water for 2 hours or overnight. Drain.

2. In a medium soup pot, heat the oil over medium-high heat and sauté the onion, carrots, celery, and soy bacon, if using, until onion is translucent, about 3 minutes.

3. Add the garlic and sauté for 1 more minute. Lower the heat and add the peppercorns, bay leaf, split peas, stock, and soy milk.

4. Reduce the heat and simmer for 1 hour. Add salt and taste for seasoning. Remove the bay leaf.

SERVES 6

Calories	Total Protein	Soy Protein	Carbohydrate	Fat	Cholesterol	Fiber	Sodium
140	8 g	1 g	19 g	4 g	0 mg	5 g	39 mg

Information is for a 1⅓-cup serving.

Soybean Minestrone

Each region of Italy—some say every household in every region!—has its own version of vegetable soup. Loaded with garlic and pasta, this southern Italian–inspired version incorporates soybeans instead of the usual white beans, which give the soup more texture along with higher protein.

2 tablespoons olive oil
1 medium onion, chopped
2 celery stalks, chopped
1 medium leek, chopped, white and
  green parts
3 garlic cloves, minced
3 plum tomatoes, coarsely chopped
8 cups Vegetable Stock (page 120)

2 sprigs of fresh oregano, stems
  removed
1 10-ounce package frozen peas
1 14-ounce can cooked soybeans
8 ounces small elbow macaroni
Salt and pepper to taste
6 fresh basil leaves, shredded

1. Heat the oil in a large skillet over medium heat and sauté the onion, celery, and leek for 5 minutes, until soft. Add the garlic and sauté for 30 seconds more.

2. Add the tomatoes, stock, oregano, peas, and soybeans and simmer for 15 minutes.

3. Add the macaroni, salt, and pepper and continue to cook for 20 minutes, until macaroni is al dente. Stir in the basil and serve at once.

SERVES 6

Calories	Total Protein	Soy Protein	Carbohydrate	Fat	Cholesterol	Fiber	Sodium
213	10 g	5 g	27 g	8 g	0 mg	3 g	154 mg

Information is for a 2-cup serving.

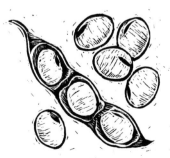

Chilled Mango Cantaloupe Soy Soup

It's a Scandinavian tradition to serve refreshing, chilled fruit soups on sunny midsummer days. This one makes a great starter or a wholesome between-meal treat. There's no cooking involved, which means it is that much easier to keep your cool. You can find mango juice in most health food stores, but if it's not available, an equal quantity of pineapple juice is a perfect substitute.

> 1 whole cantaloupe, plus another half cantaloupe for garnish
> 2 cups low-fat soy milk
> 1 cup mango juice
> 6 to 8 sprigs of mint

1. Cut the whole cantaloupe in half, scoop out seeds, and cut flesh into chunks. Put in a food processor or blender with the soy milk and mango juice. Process until the mixture is smooth. Transfer to a large bowl and chill for at least 2 hours, but no more than 24 hours.
2. With a 1-inch melon baller, make approximately 24 balls from the remaining half-cantaloupe.
3. Divide the soup among 6 bowls and garnish each serving with melon balls and mint sprigs.

SERVES 6

Calories	Total Protein	Soy Protein	Carbohydrate	Fat	Cholesterol	Fiber	Sodium
65	2.5 g	2.5 g	12 g	1.5 g	0 mg	2 g	15 mg

Information is for a 1-cup serving.

Chilled Tofu Peach Soup

Another Scandinavian-style treat, this luscious soup is at its best when you use ripe, juicy summer peaches. Tofu gives the refreshing fruit puree extra creaminess. It's a great starter or a perfect light meal on a sweltering hot day.

6 ripe, medium peaches

2 pounds low-fat silken, firm tofu

1 cup orange juice

1 cup papaya juice

2 sprigs of mint

1. Peel the peaches by blanching them in boiling water for a minute, then plunging them into a bowl of ice water. Using a sharp paring knife, remove the skins and slice the peaches.

2. Place the peaches in a food processor or blender jar and add the tofu and fruit juices. Blend the mixture until it is smooth.

3. Transfer to a large bowl and chill for at least 2 hours, but no longer than 24 hours.

4. Serve cold, garnished with mint leaves.

SERVES 6

Calories	Total Protein	Soy Protein	Carbohydrate	Fat	Cholesterol	Fiber	Sodium
146	10 g	10 g	17 g	6 g	0 mg	2 g	10 mg

Information is for a 1-cup serving.

Soy Vichyssoise

Vichyssoise—the classic French pureed leek and potato soup—is usually loaded with cream. You won't miss its absence in this soy version, which, like the original, can be served hot or cold.

> 2 medium leeks
> 2 large russet potatoes
> 1 tablespoon vegetable oil
> 1 medium white onion, chopped
> 6 cups Vegetable Stock (page 120)
> 1 cup soy milk
> ¼ teaspoon salt
> ¼ teaspoon white pepper
> ⅛ teaspoon ground nutmeg

1. Wash the leeks carefully and slice the white parts into half-inch slices. Shred the tender green parts very fine, set in a steamer basket over boiling water, and steam for 3 minutes. Set aside for garnish. Peel and dice the potatoes and place them in a bowl of cold water.

2. Heat the oil in a large pot over medium-high heat and sauté the leeks and onion until the onion is translucent, about 5 minutes.

3. Drain the potatoes and add them to the pot along with the stock. Bring to a boil and reduce the heat to low. Simmer, covered, for 30 minutes.

4. Stir in the soy milk, salt, pepper, and nutmeg. Continue to cook for 10 minutes.

5. Remove 3 cups of the soup and place in a food processor or blender. Blend until smooth and return the puree to the pot.

6. Serve the soup hot or cold. Garnish with the reserved leek greens.

SERVES 6

Calories	Total Protein	Soy Protein	Carbohydrate	Fat	Cholesterol	Fiber	Sodium
88	2.5 g	1 g	13.5 g	3 g	0 mg	2 g	104 mg

Information is for a 1½-cup serving.

Chilled Cream of Apple and Potato Soup

You may think this is an odd combination, but after you've tasted it you'll know it's a natural. In a rich leek and potato base, apples provide a hint of sweetness, while the mint and lemon juice add balance. Serve cold.

3 large red potatoes

4 medium Red Delicious apples

2 tablespoons vegetable oil

1 medium leek, sliced, white part only

1 small onion, chopped

2 celery stalks, sliced

2 garlic cloves, minced

6 cups quarts Vegetable Stock (page 120)

1 cup soy milk

2 teaspoons lemon juice

6 sprigs of mint

1. Peel and chop the potatoes. Peel, core, and chop 3 of the apples and set aside.

2. Heat the oil in a large saucepan over high heat and sauté the leek, onion, and celery for 5 minutes, until soft. Do not let them brown.

3. Lower the heat to medium and add the garlic, sautéing for 15 seconds.

4. Add the chopped potatoes, apples, and stock and bring to a boil. Lower the heat and simmer for 30 minutes, until all ingredients are very soft.

5. Remove the soup from the heat, let cool slightly, and puree in a food processor or blender. Add the soy milk, blend again, and chill for at least 1 hour. Meanwhile, quarter, core, and thinly slice the remaining apple. Toss the slices with a little lemon juice to keep them from turning brown. Serve the soup garnished with apple slices and mint.

SERVES 6

Calories	Total Protein	Soy Protein	Carbohydrate	Fat	Cholesterol	Fiber	Sodium
198	3.3 g	3.3 g	36 g	6 g	0 mg	6 g	20 mg

Information is for a 1½-cup serving.

Soy Sausage Potato Chowder

Traditional chowders are chunky meat, fish, or vegetable soups, given hearty flavor with salt pork or bacon. Most of them also contain milk, which gives them their familiar richness. You can easily replace these ingredients with soy products without affecting the taste or texture. In my version of a classic potato chowder, soy sausage takes the place of the traditional bacon or salt pork, and soy milk adds creaminess. You'll think you're in New England.

3 large russet potatoes

1 tablespoon vegetable oil

3 ounces ground soy sausage

1 small onion, chopped

1 celery stalk, chopped

3 cups Vegetable Stock (page 120)

2 cups soy milk

1 teaspoon salt

¼ teaspoon white pepper

¼ cup chopped parsley, for garnish

1. Peel the potatoes, dice them, and place in a bowl of cold water to keep them from turning brown.

2. Heat the oil in a large pot over medium-high heat and crumble the sausage into it. Add the onion and celery and sauté until the onion is translucent, about 5 minutes. Do not brown the onion.

3. Add the potatoes and stock. Bring the mixture to a boil and reduce the heat to low. Simmer for 30 minutes, until vegetables are very soft.

4. Add the soy milk, salt, and pepper, and simmer for 20 more minutes.

5. Serve hot, garnished with fresh parsley.

SERVES 6 TO 8

Calories	Total Protein	Soy Protein	Carbohydrate	Fat	Cholesterol	Fiber	Sodium
107	5 g	5 g	15 g	3 g	0 mg	2 g	310 mg

Information is for a 1-cup serving.

Tofu Corn Chowder

Corn chowder is another New England classic. Soy milk gives this soup a rich texture and the added chunks of tofu make it a nutritious meal in itself. This is as lovely to look at as it is to eat, with red and green peppers and yellow corn kernels floating in a creamy base.

1 tablespoon vegetable oil

1 large white onion, chopped

1 small red bell pepper, seeded and chopped

1 small green bell pepper, seeded and chopped

1 10-ounce package frozen corn, thawed

2 cups Vegetable Stock (page 120)

4 medium red potatoes, diced

1½ cups soy milk

1½ pounds firm tofu, cubed

1 teaspoon salt

½ teaspoon black pepper

¼ cup chopped parsley

1. Heat the oil in a medium saucepan over high heat and sauté the onion, peppers, and corn until the onion is translucent, about 5 minutes.

2. Add the stock and potatoes and bring to a boil. Reduce the heat to a simmer and cook for 15 minutes, until vegetables are very soft.

3. Add the soy milk and tofu and simmer for another 15 minutes. Season with salt and pepper. Serve immediately, garnished with parsley.

SERVES 6

Calories	Total Protein	Soy Protein	Carbohydrate	Fat	Cholesterol	Fiber	Sodium
150	10 g	10 g	15 g	6 g	0 mg	2 g	282 mg

Information is for a 1-cup serving.

Soybean Chili

In this medium-spicy chili, soybeans take the place of the kidney beans usually used. The flavor remains the same, but the texture is chewier than chili made with mushier beans. This chili makes a hearty main course, served over brown rice and topped with a little shredded soy jack cheese. It's also delicious as a bean dip or burrito filling. It freezes well for up to three months.

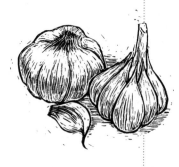

1 tablespoon olive oil
2 medium onions, chopped
6 garlic cloves, minced
1 14½-ounce can chopped tomatoes, including juice
1 tablespoon dried oregano
1 tablespoon ground cumin
1 tablespoon chili powder
2 15-ounce cans cooked soybeans or 2 cups cooked dried soybeans (page 62)

1. Heat the oil in a large pot over medium-high heat and sauté the onions and garlic until they are translucent, about 5 minutes. Add the tomatoes and sauté for 3 to 4 more minutes.

2. Stir in the oregano, cumin, and chili powder, sautéing for 2 to 3 minutes more.

3. Add the soybeans and bring the mixture to a boil. Reduce the heat to low and simmer for 45 minutes. (The chili can be made a day or two ahead and reheated.)

SERVES 6

Calories	Total Protein	Soy Protein	Carbohydrate	Fat	Cholesterol	Fiber	Sodium
117	8 g	8 g	15 g	4 g	0 mg	2 g	11 mg

Information is for a 1-cup serving.

Black Bean Chili with Tempeh

This Southwestern-style chili adds tempeh to black beans for a nutritional boost. It is on the mild side; if you like it hot, just double the amount of chili powder. Soy Cheese Corn Bread (page 99) makes the perfect accompaniment. This recipe will keep for several days in the refrigerator or up to three months in the freezer. I like to double it and have some on hand for busy weeks or unexpected guests.

1 tablespoon vegetable oil

2 medium onions, chopped

6 garlic cloves, minced

1 14½-ounce can chopped tomatoes, including juices

1 tablespoon dried oregano

1 tablespoon ground cumin

1 tablespoon chili powder

2 15-ounce cans black beans, drained

8 ounces tempeh, crumbled

1 cup soy sour cream (optional)

1. Heat the oil in a large saucepan over medium-high heat and sauté the onions and garlic until the onions are translucent, about 5 minutes. Add the tomatoes and continue cooking for 3 to 4 more minutes.

2. Stir in the oregano, cumin, and chili powder, sautéing for 2 to 3 minutes more.

3. Add the black beans, bring to a boil, and reduce the heat to low.

4. Stir in the tempeh and simmer, covered, for 1 hour. Serve hot, topped with a dollop of soy sour cream, if desired.

SERVES 6

Calories	Total Protein	Soy Protein	Carbohydrate	Fat	Cholesterol	Fiber	Sodium
207	13 g	6 g	30 g	4.5 g	0 mg	7.4 g	9 mg

Information is for a 1¼-cup serving.

Espagnole Sauce

½ cup soy sauce
½ cup dry red wine
2 cups Vegetable Stock
   (page 120)
2 cups soy milk
½ cup tomato paste
3 tablespoons vegetable oil
1 medium shallot, chopped
1 small onion, chopped
1 medium carrot, chopped
4 large white mushrooms,
   chopped
3 garlic cloves, finely
   minced
2 tablespoons all-purpose
   flour
2 bay leaves
1 teaspoon dried thyme
1 teaspoon dried rosemary
¼ cup chopped parsley
½ teaspoon black pepper

1. In a mixing bowl, combine the soy sauce, wine, stock, soy milk, and tomato paste, and mix thoroughly. Set aside.
2. Heat the vegetable oil in a saucepan over high heat, and sauté the shallot, onion, carrot, and mushrooms for 3 minutes. Add the garlic and sauté for 1 more minute.

Hearty Tofu Stew

Chunks of potatoes, carrots, leeks, and delicious mushrooms, simmering in a rich vegetable stock make this filling stew a wonderful choice for a cool night. It gets its flavor from the addition of espagnole sauce, a dense reduction of vegetables and herbs. Because espagnole sauce is so useful and freezes perfectly, I always have a quantity in my freezer. That makes this mouthwatering stew is a snap to prepare, though it tastes as if it took all day. I like to serve it over wide noodles or brown rice, or just piping hot in a mug.

1 large onion
1 medium leek
3 large carrots
3 celery stalks
1 large green bell pepper
6 large white mushrooms
2 tablespoons vegetable oil
3 garlic cloves, minced

3 cups Vegetable Stock (page 120)
2 cups Espagnole Sauce (see sidebar)
2 medium red potatoes, cut into large chunks
1 10-ounce package frozen corn
1½ pounds firm tofu, cubed
Salt and pepper to taste

1. Cut the onion, leek, carrots, celery, green pepper, and mushrooms into large chunks. Heat the oil in a large pot over high heat and sauté the cut vegetables for 5 minutes. Lower the heat and add the garlic, cooking for 30 more seconds.

2. Add the stock, espagnole sauce, potatoes, and corn and simmer, covered, for 30 minutes. Add the tofu cubes, and simmer another 15 minutes. Season with salt and pepper.

SERVES 6

Calories	Total Protein	Soy Protein	Carbohydrate	Fat	Cholesterol	Fiber	Sodium
418	23.5 g	18 g	49 g	17 g	0 mg	10 g	752 mg

Information is for a 1½-cup serving.

Country Soy Sausage Stew

Imagine an aromatic French beef stew with shallots, tomatoes, carrots, garlic, and marjoram. Now replace the chunks of beef with ground soy sausage and you'll have an idea of what this dish is like. This is fabulous over Soy Polenta (page 184) or wide noodles, accompanied by Mixed Baby Greens with Mustard Tarragon Soy Vinaigrette (page 50).

2 tablespoons vegetable oil

2 14-ounce packages beef-flavored soy sausage

½ small onion, chopped

1 small shallot, chopped

2 celery stalks, chopped

3 large carrots, chopped

3 garlic cloves, minced

6 medium tomatoes, chopped, or 1 14 ½-ounce can diced tomatoes

1 bay leaf, crushed

2 teaspoons dried tarragon

2 teaspoons dried marjoram

1 teaspoon dried sage

4 cups Vegetable Stock (page 120)

¼ teaspoon salt

¼ teaspoon pepper

8 ounces soy garlic–and–herb cheese, grated

1. Heat the oil in a stockpot over medium-high heat and sauté the sausage, onion, shallot, celery, and carrots for 5 minutes, stirring frequently to prevent sticking. Add the garlic and sauté for 1 more minute.

2. Add the tomatoes, herbs, and a small amount of stock. Sauté for 1 minute, and add the remaining stock, the salt, and pepper. Simmer for 1 hour. Spoon into bowls and sprinkle soy garlic–and–herb cheese on top.

SERVES 8

Calories	Total Protein	Soy Protein	Carbohydrate	Fat	Cholesterol	Fiber	Sodium
268	26 g	25 g	23 g	7 g	0 mg	2.5 g	650 mg

Information is for a 1½-cup serving.

3. Lower the heat and add the flour. Continue to cook until the mixture is slightly browned. Stir in herbs and pepper.

4. Add the soy sauce mixture to the vegetables and stir until well blended. Cover and simmer for 30 minutes. Strain the sauce through a fine mesh before serving.

MAKES 6 CUPS OF SAUCE

Calories: 135, Total Protein: 6 g,	
Soy Protein: 2 g, Carbohydrate: 19 g,	
Fat: 22 g, Cholesterol: 0 mg,	
Fiber: 9 g, Sodium: 706 mg	

Information is for a ¼-cup serving.

six

main dishes

What's for dinner? In the following pages, you'll find mouthwatering soy-centered entrees: a spicy curry inspired by India; a rich, tomato-sauced cacciatore from Italy; a fragrant Mexican mole sauce; grilled tempeh kabobs; a comforting, down-home pot pie; a spicy Szechuan stir-fry; a saffron-infused Spanish paella; a jazzy Cajun jambalaya.

Clearly, there's no cuisine, no style of cooking, no flavor that can't showcase soy. Protein-packed tofu, tempeh, and meat analogs stand in deliciously for chicken, fish, and meats in these hearty main dishes. The recipes are grouped according to main ingredient: in the tofu section, for example, you'll find aromatic Tofu with Mexican Mole Sauce; the tempeh section features easy Grilled Tempeh with Barbecue Sauce, and the soy sausage section stars all-American Soy Meat Loaf and rich Soy Hungarian Goulash.

For the most part, handling soy ingredients in these main dishes is remarkably similar to handling regular meats and poultry. For example, the Garden Kabobs with Orange Sauce features marinated tempeh and vegetables threaded on a skewer and grilled exactly as you would chunks of chicken or beef. One thing to keep in mind is that soy meat analogs have very little fat and therefore tend to stick to the pan when browning. For best results, use nonstick pans, add a little soybean or olive oil, and stir constantly when cooking.

Main courses using soy products are the perfect place to let your creativity soar. For instance, a cooking class recently inspired me to try substituting tempeh for beef in one classic dish; the result was the fabulous Spinach Tempeh in Pastry Pockets: flaky puff pastry encasing delectable bundles of tempeh, spinach, scallions, and walnuts. I re-created my grandmother's incredible stuffed cabbage with a savory soy-sausage filling that actually improves upon the original! All these easy, healthful, and satisfying main courses are destined to become family classics.

Papaya Pear Chutney

1 large papaya, peeled, seeded, and diced
2 large Bosc pears, cored and diced
1 small red onion, chopped
¼ cup brown sugar
1 cup orange juice
¼ teaspoon salt
⅛ teaspoon white pepper
¼ teaspoon ground cinnamon
⅛ teaspoon ground cloves
¼ teaspoon ground nutmeg
¼ teaspoon ground ginger
4 sprigs of mint, chopped
¼ cup chopped cilantro

1. Place the papaya, pears, onion, and brown sugar in a medium saucepan. Add the orange juice and bring to a boil over high heat.
2. When the sugar is dissolved, after about 3 minutes, reduce the heat and add the salt, pepper, cinnamon, cloves, nutmeg, and ginger. Simmer for 10 minutes.
3. Add the mint and cilantro, cover, and cook for 5 minutes more, or until the liquid has reduced to a syrupy consistency. Remove from the heat and transfer to a bowl to cool. The chutney can be made and refrigerated several days in advance. It will keep, well sealed, in the refrigerator for up to 2 weeks.

Tofu with Mexican Mole Sauce

The "secret ingredient" in this aromatic dish is, surprisingly, unsweetened cocoa powder. Chicken or turkey in a rich brown mole sauce is a favorite festival dish for Mexicans, who learned the cocoa trick from their Aztec ancestors. The thick, fragrant sauce works just as well with slices of tofu as it does with poultry. The cocoa powder makes the sauce dark and glossy; combined with the cinnamon, it adds a delectable, spicy bouquet. Serve this with Spanish Brown Rice Pilaf (page 182).

1 tablespoon olive oil
2 medium onions, minced
1 small green bell pepper, minced
3 garlic cloves, minced
5 ripe, medium tomatoes, diced
2 dried mild chilies, soaked in water to cover for 1 hour and finely minced
1 teaspoon ground cinnamon
¼ teaspoon dried thyme
2 cups Vegetable Stock (page 120)
¼ cup chopped cilantro
⅓ cup unsweetened cocoa powder
1 teaspoon salt
2 tablespoons vegetable oil
3 pounds firm tofu, each pound cut into 6 even slices

1. Heat the olive oil in a large saucepan over high heat and sauté the onions and green pepper until the onions are browned, about 8 minutes. Add the garlic and sauté for 30 more seconds.
2. Lower the heat to medium-low and add the tomatoes, chilies, cinnamon, and thyme. Stir until the mixture reaches the consistency of a paste, about 5 more minutes.
3. Add the stock and cilantro, and simmer on very low heat for 30 minutes. Stir in the cocoa until it is combined and simmer for another 10 minutes. Season with salt.
4. Heat the vegetable oil in a skillet over medium-high heat and add the tofu, lightly browning both sides, about 3 minutes on each side.
5. Place 3 slices of tofu on each of 6 plates and cover evenly with mole sauce.

SERVES 6

Calories	Total Protein	Soy Protein	Carbohydrate	Fat	Cholesterol	Fiber	Sodium
277	21 g	18 g	15 g	16 g	0 mg	4 g	397 mg

Information is for a 3-slice serving.

the whole soy cookbook

Tofu Curry with Papaya Pear Chutney

MAKES 4 CUPS

The vibrant flavors of curry, cumin, cardamom, ginger, and garlic are absorbed by cubes of velvety tofu and sweet apple in this luscious Indian-style dish. The sweet-and-sour chutney provides the perfect balance for the spiciness of the dish. The tofu cubes and brown rice provide complete protein. For a real taste of India, serve this accompanied by Cucumber Raita (page 46) and Garlic naan, an Indian bread readily available in specialty markets.

Calories: 35, Total Protein: 0 g,	
Soy Protein: 0 g, Carbohydrate: 8.8 g,	
Fat: 0 g, Cholesterol: 0 mg, Fiber: 1 g,	
Sodium: 35 mg	

Information is for a 2-tablespoon serving.

8 ounces plain soy yogurt

1 tablespoon curry powder

1 teaspoon ground cumin

½ teaspoon crushed red pepper

1 1-inch piece fresh ginger, minced

1 teaspoon ground cardamom

1½ tablespoons olive oil

1 large onion, diced

½ pound button mushrooms, sliced

1 large Granny Smith apple, cored and diced

2½ pounds firm tofu, cut into 1-inch cubes

½ cup apple juice

2 cups cooked brown rice

½ small bunch cilantro

1 cup Papaya Pear Chutney (see sidebar)

1. In a food processor or blender, blend together the yogurt, curry, cumin, red pepper, ginger, and cardamom and set aside.

2. Heat the olive oil in a large saucepan over high heat and sauté the onion and mushrooms until the onion is translucent, 3 to 5 minutes. Add the diced apple and sauté until softened, about 3 more minutes.

3. Stir in the soy yogurt mixture and the tofu cubes. Simmer, partially covered, over very low heat for 30 minutes. Add small amounts of apple juice if the curry seems too thick.

4. Serve immediately over the rice, garnished with fresh cilantro sprigs. Pass chutney on the side.

SERVES 6

Calories	Total Protein	Soy Protein	Carbohydrate	Fat	Cholesterol	Fiber	Sodium
240	13 g	12 g	27 g	10 g	0 mg	3.1 g	20 mg

Information is for a 1½-cup serving, including rice and chutney.

Tofu Cacciatore

The classic dish is chicken cacciatore: breasts of chicken smothered in chunky tomato sauce. In my soy rendition, the aromatic, garlicky sauce brings out the best in tofu. Serve with rice or flat noodles, a bold red wine, and plenty of crusty bread to mop up the hearty sauce. For a thoroughly Italian meal, finish with Soy Tiramisù (page 204) or coffee and Orange-Walnut Biscotti (page 193).

3 pounds firm tofu

⅓ cup olive oil

¾ pound fresh mushrooms, sliced

1 small yellow onion, finely chopped

1 medium shallot, minced

1 celery stalk, finely chopped

3 garlic cloves, minced

¾ cup dry red wine

1⅓ cups Vegetable Stock (page 120)

1 tablespoon Italian seasoning

1 pound ripe tomatoes, coarsely chopped, or 1 14-ounce can diced tomatoes

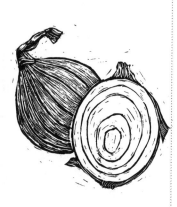

1. Preheat the broiler. Slice each pound of tofu into 6 slices and place on baking sheets. Brush lightly with olive oil and broil for about 5 minutes. Set aside.

2. Heat 1 tablespoon of the remaining olive oil in a large skillet over medium heat and sauté the mushrooms until they are softened, about 5 minutes. Remove mushrooms and set aside.

3. In the same pan, over high heat, sauté the onion, shallot, and celery in an additional tablespoon of olive oil for 3 minutes. Add the garlic and cook for 1 more minute.

4. Reduce the heat and add the wine. When wine evaporates, add the stock and Italian seasoning, turn heat up to medium, and let the mixture cook until it is reduced by half, about 30 minutes.

5. Return the mushrooms to the pan and add the tomatoes. Simmer for 5 minutes or until tomatoes are heated thoroughly. Place tofu on a platter and cover with sauce.

SERVES 6

Calories	Total Protein	Soy Protein	Carbohydrate	Fat	Cholesterol	Fiber	Sodium
450	38 g	36 g	20 g	17 g	0 mg	6 g	159 mg

Information is for 1 3-slice serving.

Broiled Tofu with Five-Onion Sauce

There are many different kinds of onion, each with a subtle taste of its own. This recipe blends the flavors of five varieties of onion, which are caramelized over low heat so they become sweet and rich tasting. The aromatic sauce is spooned over broiled tofu. Note: if you can't find Maui onions, you can substitute any other sweet onion, such as Vidalia or Walla Walla.

2 pounds firm tofu
2 tablespoons olive oil
2 tablespoons vegetable oil
1 small Maui onion, chopped
1 medium yellow onion, chopped
1 medium red onion, chopped
1 medium leek, white and tender
   green parts, chopped

1 medium shallot, chopped
1 tablespoon unbleached all-
   purpose flour
¼ teaspoon dried sage
1 cup Vegetable Stock (page 120)
Salt and pepper to taste

1. Preheat the broiler.
2. Cut the tofu into 12 even squares. Place on a cookie sheet and brush lightly with the olive oil. Broil the tofu for 10 minutes or until the top browns slightly. Remove from the heat.
3. Heat the vegetable oil in a saucepan over medium-high heat and add the onions, leek, and shallot. Sauté until onions start to brown, about 5 minutes, and lower heat.
4. Stir in the flour and sage and cook, stirring frequently, until the onions are caramelized, about 10 minutes. Add the stock and cook for 5 more minutes. Season with salt and pepper and remove from heat.
5. Place 2 pieces of tofu on each of 6 dinner plates and spoon ⅓ cup of onion sauce over each.

SERVES 6

Calories	Total Protein	Soy Protein	Carbohydrate	Fat	Cholesterol	Fiber	Sodium
313	25 g	25 g	18 g	18 g	0 mg	4.5 g	34 mg

Information is for a 2-piece serving.

Herbed Tofu Chapati Wraps

These are sophisticated bundles of tofu and tempeh, sandwiched with a piquant herb spread and glazed with a flavorful sauce. Chapati are thin Indian griddle breads. You can usually find them in larger markets or specialty stores, but large whole wheat tortillas work just as well if chapati are unavailable. Don't be dismayed by the length of this recipe. Both the herb paste and the sauce can be made in advance and frozen until ready to use, and the leftovers of both are useful in other dishes. Herb paste is a little like pesto: it makes a tasty spread for focaccia or an ingredient in dips or salad dressings.

Herb Paste

1 cup fresh basil leaves

¾ cup cilantro leaves

¼ cup fresh thyme leaves

½ cup fresh dill

3 garlic cloves

3 tablespoons olive oil

1½ pounds tempeh

14 ounces firm tofu

6 whole wheat chapati

2 cups Espagnole Sauce (page 136)

1. Place the basil, cilantro, thyme, dill, garlic, and olive oil in a blender container or food processor and process until smooth. Reserve ½ cup for this recipe. (Makes 1½ cups; freeze the remainder for future use.)

2. Preheat the oven to 350°F.

3. Slice the tempeh cakes in half. In a steamer basket set over boiling water, steam the 6 pieces of tempeh for 5 minutes, or until soft. Cut the tofu into 6 even slices.

4. Spread 1 tablespoon of herb paste in the middle of a whole wheat chapati. Place a slice of tempeh over the herb paste and a slice of tofu on top of that. Fold the chapati, enchilada style, tucking the ends under. Repeat the process for remaining 5 chapatis.

5. Place the chapati wraps in an ovenproof dish and cover with foil. Bake for 15 minutes. Meanwhile, heat the sauce.

6. Spoon ⅓ cup sauce in the center of each of 6 plates and put a chapati wrap in the middle, or serve buffet style, on a warm platter, with the warm sauce on the side.

SERVES 6

Calories	Total Protein	Soy Protein	Carbohydrate	Fat	Cholesterol	Fiber	Sodium
550	34 g	33 g	60 g	22 g	0 mg	9 g	706 mg

Information is for 1 chapati wrap.

Maui Tofu

Cubes of tofu mingle with colorful red and green peppers in this delicious stir-fry. The Hawaiian-style sauce, incorporating sweet pineapple, zingy ginger, and salty soy sauce, beautifully complements the velvety tofu. Serve over a bed of hot rice.

2 tablespoons toasted sesame oil
2 teaspoons vegetable oil
¼ cup soy sauce
1 medium onion, sliced
1 medium green bell pepper, seeded and sliced
1 medium red bell pepper, seeded and sliced

2 garlic cloves, minced
1 1-inch piece fresh ginger, grated
1 cup chopped pineapple, with juices
1 cup Vegetable Stock (page 120)
1 pound extra-firm tofu, cubed
¼ head green cabbage, shredded
3 cups cooked rice

1. Heat the sesame oil, vegetable oil, and soy sauce over high heat in a large saucepan or wok and sauté the onion and peppers for 5 minutes.
2. Add the garlic and ginger, cooking for 1 more minute.
3. Add the pineapple, stock, and tofu and simmer for 15 minutes. Toss in the shredded cabbage and serve over rice immediately.

SERVES 6

Calories	Total Protein	Soy Protein	Carbohydrate	Fat	Cholesterol	Fiber	Sodium
192	13 g	6 g	12 g	12 g	0 mg	3 g	708 mg

Information is for a 1-cup serving, including a ½-cup of rice.

Broiled Tofu with Braised Beans and Vegetables

Picture a bed of colorful yellow squash and zucchini sticks. On it rests a lightly browned slice of tofu, crowned with a delicious mixture of fresh herbs, tomatoes, and braised beans. This dish is as pretty to look at as it is delicious to eat! When I serve this to dinner guests, I like to start with Soy Vichyssoise (page 130) and complete the meal with luscious Tofu Chocolate Mousse (page 191).

2 tablespoons vegetable oil

1 medium leek, white part only, chopped

⅓ cup dry sherry

1½ tablespoons chopped fresh tarragon

1½ tablespoons chopped parsley

2¼ cups Vegetable Stock (page 120)

2 14-ounce cans soybeans, drained

4 plum tomatoes, coarsely chopped

Salt and pepper, to taste

2 pounds firm tofu

2 tablespoons olive oil

1 medium zucchini, cut into long matchsticks

2 medium yellow squash, cut into long matchsticks

1. In a saucepan, heat the vegetable oil over medium heat. Add the leek and sauté for 1 minute. Stir in the sherry and cook for 1 minute or until the liquid has reduced slightly.

2. Add the herbs and 2 cups of the stock and bring the mixture to a boil. Add the beans, reduce the heat to low and simmer for 20 minutes, stirring occasionally. Add the tomatoes, salt, and pepper and heat thoroughly. Keep warm while preparing the tofu.

3. Preheat the broiler. Slice the tofu into 12 even square pieces. Place on a baking sheet and brush with olive oil. Broil for 8 to 10 minutes, or until the tofu browns evenly. Remove and set aside.

4. In a medium skillet, heat the remaining ¼ cup stock over medium-high heat. Add the zucchini and yellow squash and stir for 3 to 5 minutes, until the vegetable sticks are just tender.

5. Divide the vegetables among 6 plates, arranging them in a circle. Place the tofu slices on top and cover with the soybean mixture. Serve immediately.

SERVES 6

Calories	Total Protein	Soy Protein	Carbohydrate	Fat	Cholesterol	Fiber	Sodium
534	38 g	36 g	24 g	30 g	0 mg	10 g	177 mg

Information is for a 2-slice serving.

Tofu Pot Pie

This savory pot pie is as comforting as Grandma's original but a lot easier to make, thanks to ready-made pie crust and tofu. A mixed green salad with Creamy Herb Dressing (page 72) completes the meal.

1 cup Vegetable Stock (page 120)

1 cup soy milk

1 teaspoon poultry seasoning

½ teaspoon white pepper

4 large carrots, peeled and diced

2 medium russet potatoes, peeled and diced

¼ teaspoon salt

2 cups frozen pearl onions

2 cups frozen peas

1 pound firm tofu, cubed

Pie crust dough for 2 double-crust 8-inch pies (page 201) or 4 ready-made crusts

1. Preheat the oven to 375°F.

2. In a large saucepan, combine the stock, soy milk, poultry seasoning, and pepper and bring to a boil. Add the carrots, potatoes, and salt and bring to a second boil. Reduce the heat and simmer for 5 minutes.

3. Add the onions, peas, and tofu and simmer, covered, another 5 minutes.

4. Line two 8-inch pie dishes with a pie crust each. Pour the vegetable-tofu mixture into the shells and top with the remaining 2 pie crusts. Crimp the edges decoratively and cut 3 slashes in the top of each pie.

5. Bake for 30 minutes, or until lightly browned. Serve immediately. (Freeze one pie, tightly wrapped, for future use, if desired.)

MAKES 2 PIES, EACH SERVING 6

Calories	Total Protein	Soy Protein	Carbohydrate	Fat	Cholesterol	Fiber	Sodium
323	11 g	9 g	35 g	17 g	0 mg	4.2 g	342 mg

Information is per serving.

Kung Pao Tempeh

If you have tempeh and a little fresh ginger in your refrigerator, it's easier to cook Chinese food yourself than it is to order out. You'll more than likely already have in your cupboard all the other ingredients for this adaptation of a Szechuan restaurant favorite. Kung Pao usually refers to chicken in a peanut sauce, but tempeh works beautifully in place of poultry. It holds its shape just as well, is easier to store and handle, and is much quicker to cook. Serve this over white rice.

¼ cup low-sodium soy sauce

¼ cup white wine vinegar

½ cup dry sherry

1⅓ cups Vegetable Stock (page 120)

2 tablespoons honey

1 pound tempeh

1 tablespoon cornstarch

1 tablespoon salt

½ teaspoon white pepper

3 tablespoons roasted sesame oil

1 tablespoon vegetable oil

1 dried mild chili pepper, crushed, or 1 teaspoon crushed red pepper

6 garlic cloves, minced

1 2-inch piece fresh ginger, minced

½ cup smooth low-sodium peanut butter

½ cup soy milk

4 scallions, sliced, green and white parts

3 cups hot cooked white rice

1. Whisk together the soy sauce, vinegar, ¼ cup sherry, the stock, and honey and set aside.

2. Cut the tempeh into small squares and, in a steamer basket set over boiling water, steam for 5 minutes.

3. In a medium mixing bowl, combine the remaining ¼ cup sherry, the cornstarch, salt, pepper, and sesame oil. Add the tempeh and let marinate while sautéing the remaining ingredients.

4. Heat the vegetable oil in a skillet over medium heat and cook the chili pepper for one minute, being careful not to burn it. Lower the heat, add the garlic and ginger, and cook for 30 seconds.

5. Stir in the peanut butter, soy milk, and soy sauce mixture. Add the tempeh along with its marinade and simmer over very low heat for 10 minutes. Serve over rice immediately, garnished with scallions.

SERVES 6

Calories	Total Protein	Soy Protein	Carbohydrate	Fat	Cholesterol	Fiber	Sodium
454	19.5 g	15 g	61 g	27 g	0 mg	7 g	1796 mg

Information is for a 1-cup serving.

Tempeh Pepper "Steak"

Pepper steak—strips of beef round steak stir-fried with colorful red and green peppers in a ginger sauce—is one of the most familiar dishes on a traditional Chinese menu. Unfortunately, round steak can often be tough and chewy. You'll never have that problem with healthful tempeh. Serve this flavorful stir-fry with white rice.

1 pound tempeh

1 tablespoon vegetable oil

1 tablespoon roasted sesame oil

4 garlic cloves, minced

1 medium onion, sliced

1 medium red bell pepper, sliced

1 medium green bell pepper, sliced

1 ½-inch piece fresh ginger, minced

2 tablespoons low-sodium soy sauce

3 cups hot cooked rice

1. In a large pot, set a steamer basket over boiling water. Dice the tempeh into 1-inch cubes and steam, covered, for 5 minutes or until soft. Set aside.

2. In a saucepan, heat the vegetable and sesame oils over medium-high heat, and sauté the garlic for 15 seconds. Add the sliced onion and red and green peppers, and stir-fry for 3 to 4 minutes.

3. Stir in the ginger and soy sauce and add the steamed tempeh. Stir-fry for 3 more minutes.

4. Serve immediately over hot rice.

SERVES 6

Calories	Total Protein	Soy Protein	Carbohydrate	Fat	Cholesterol	Fiber	Sodium
342	17.5 g	14 g	46 g	11 g	0 mg	4.5 g	206 mg

Information is for a 1-cup serving, including ½-cup of rice.

Szechuan Tempeh

Chinese cuisine varies widely according to the region of its origin. Of the three styles most familiar to Americans—Mandarin, Cantonese, and Szechuan—the spiciest is Szechuan. Depending on how fireproof your palate is, you can vary the quantity of black and red pepper in this stir-fry. Tempeh takes the place of the usual pork or chicken, making it not only healthier but much easier to prepare. Serve with white rice.

1 pound tempeh, at room temperature

1 medium green bell pepper

½ pound fresh mushrooms

1 medium onion

2 tablespoons peanut oil (or more if needed)

1 teaspoon ground ginger

2 tablespoons brown sugar

2 teaspoons crushed black peppercorns

1 teaspoon crushed red pepper (or less, to taste)

½ cup unsalted cashew halves

1 cup Vegetable Stock (page 120)

⅔ cup soy sauce

⅓ cup dry sherry

3 cups cooked white rice

1. Cut the tempeh into small cubes. Slice the pepper, mushrooms, and onion. Combine all three in a bowl and set aside.

2. Heat the peanut oil in a large wok or skillet over high heat and add the ginger, brown sugar, black pepper, and red pepper. Stir in the tempeh, pepper, mushrooms, onion, and the cashews.

3. Cook, stirring constantly, for 5 minutes.

4. Lower the heat to medium and add the stock, soy sauce, and sherry. Reduce the heat again and let simmer for 10 minutes. Serve over rice immediately.

SERVES 6

Calories	Total Protein	Soy Protein	Carbohydrate	Fat	Cholesterol	Fiber	Sodium
439	21 g	14 g	60 g	13 g	0 mg	46 g	620 mg

Information is for a 1-cup serving, including a ½-cup of rice.

Near Eastern Curried Tempeh

The sweetness of apricots, apples, and raisins combined with the spiciness of onions and curry powder gives this dish a definite Middle Eastern feel. For this reason, I like to serve it accompanied by Couscous and Cranberries (page 185), a delicious Arab-style dish.

1 pound tempeh

3 tablespoons vegetable oil

½ cup chopped yellow onion

1 celery stalk, chopped

½ cup apricot preserves

½ cup tomato paste

2 tablespoons curry powder

Salt

½ cup chopped Red Delicious apple

½ cup raisins

1 cup tomato juice

1. In a large pot, set a steamer basket over boiling water. Dice the tempeh into 1-inch cubes and steam, covered, for 5 minutes, or until softened.

2. In a medium skillet, heat the oil and sauté the onion and celery for 3 minutes.

3. In a separate bowl, combine the apricot preserves, tomato paste, curry powder, and salt, mixing well.

4. Mix the apple and raisins into the curry mixture. Add the curried apple mixture to the onion and celery. Stir in the tomato juice and cook over low heat for 5 minutes, stirring frequently.

5. Add the steamed tempeh cubes and continue to cook over low heat for another 15 minutes. The mixture will be very thick. Serve immediately.

SERVES 6

Calories	Total Protein	Soy Protein	Carbohydrate	Fat	Cholesterol	Fiber	Sodium
367	16.2 g	14 g	52 g	0 g	0 mg	7 g	33.5 mg

Information is for a 1-cup serving.

Tempeh Fajitas

A fajita is a flour tortilla filled with shredded, grilled, marinated meat cut with the grain, so that it shreds easily. When you order fajitas in a Mexican restaurant these days, though, you're as likely to get shrimp as the usual beef or chicken with peppers and onions. Because tempeh holds its shape when sliced into strips, it works beautifully as a substitute for meat in this favorite dish from the Oaxacan region of Mexico. Serve this with guacamole, cheese, and sour cream for topping.

12 large flour tortillas
1½ pounds tempeh, cut into
  ¼-inch-wide strips
1 small white onion
1 small red onion
1 large red bell pepper
1 large green bell pepper

2 tablespoons vegetable oil
3 garlic cloves, minced
¼ cup chopped cilantro
2 tablespoons chili powder
1 tablespoon ground cumin
Salt and pepper to taste

1. Preheat the oven to 250°F. Stack the tortillas and wrap in foil and place in the oven to warm.

2. In a steamer basket set over boiling water, steam the tempeh strips for 5 minutes and set aside in a bowl.

3. Cut the onions and bell peppers into strips, and add to the tempeh.

4. Heat the oil in a large skillet over high heat and sauté the tempeh, onions, and bell peppers until onions are translucent, about 5 minutes.

5. Lower the heat to medium and add the garlic, cilantro, chili powder, cumin, salt, and pepper. Sauté for 3 more minutes. Serve immediately with warm tortillas.

SERVES 6

Calories	Total Protein	Soy Protein	Carbohydrate	Fat	Cholesterol	Fiber	Sodium
482	27 g	21 g	59 g	17.3 g	0 mg	6.7 g	20 mg

Information is for 2 tortillas, including 1½-cups filling.

Tempeh Dijonaisse

This version of the classic French poulet à la diable *(deviled chicken breasts) works beautifully with broiled tempeh standing in for the chicken. Serve with steamed green beans and Garlic Mashed Potatoes with Soy Milk (page 55).*

1½ pounds tempeh
2 tablespoons olive oil
½ cup Dijon mustard
¼ cup honey
½ cup cider vinegar
¼ cup soy milk
3 scallions, sliced, green and white parts

1. Have all ingredients at room temperature. Preheat the broiler.

2. Halve each piece of tempeh. Brush the 6 slices with olive oil and broil for 5 minutes on each side.

3. In a medium saucepan, whisk together the mustard, honey, and cider vinegar. Cook over very low heat while the tempeh broils, adding the soy milk toward the end and stirring until it is thoroughly heated.

4. Arrange the tempeh on a platter or individual plates and pour the sauce over it. Garnish with scallion slices.

SERVES 6

Calories	Total Protein	Soy Protein	Carbohydrate	Fat	Cholesterol	Fiber	Sodium
323	22 g	21 g	32 g	13 g	0 mg	3.5 g	219 mg

Information is for a 1-slice serving.

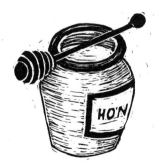

Grilled Tempeh with Barbecue Sauce

Tempeh squares hold up on the grill every bit as well as hamburger or chicken breasts. Treat the tempeh as you would a burger: serve it plain or on a whole wheat bun. Good side dishes for a summer barbecue meal include corn on the cob, baked beans, and Confetti Slaw with Tomato-Soy Yogurt Dressing (page 56).

4 pounds tempeh

Barbecue Sauce

2 tablespoons vegetable oil

1 large onion, minced

8 garlic cloves, minced

2 cups Vegetable Stock (page 120)

2 cups ketchup

½ cup molasses or honey

¼ cup low-sodium soy sauce

4 tablespoons brown mustard

½ teaspoon paprika

1 teaspoon dried thyme

⅓ cup dry sherry

1. Cut the tempeh cakes in half. In a steamer basket set over boiling water, steam them for 5 minutes.

2. Heat the oil in a large saucepan over high heat, and sauté the onion for 5 minutes. Add the garlic and sauté 1 more minute.

3. Add all of the remaining ingredients except the sherry in order, stirring constantly until they are thoroughly mixed. Lower heat and simmer the sauce for 20 minutes. Stir in the sherry and remove from the heat. Reserve 1 cup for the tempeh. (Makes 4 cups; extra sauce can be stored in the refrigerator for up to 2 weeks.)

4. Marinate the tempeh pieces in the sauce for 1 hour or as long as overnight.

5. Place tempeh on an outdoor grill or in an oven broiler, and cook on each side for 5 minutes, or just until sauce on top starts to blacken. Serve immediately and pass extra warm barbecue sauce on the side.

SERVES 8

Calories	Total Protein	Soy Protein	Carbohydrate	Fat	Cholesterol	Fiber	Sodium
323	22 g	21 g	32 g	13 g	0 mg	3.5 g	219 mg

Information is for a 1-slice serving, including 1 ounce of sauce.

Garden Kabobs with Orange Sauce

These vegetable and tempeh kabobs can be assembled a day before cooking and allowed to marinate until needed. You can cook them on an outdoor barbecue grill or broil them in the oven. Serve as a main course, on a bed of rice or Soy Cheddar Pilaf (page 183), with a green salad and toasted Soy Herb Bread (page 104).

> 1 medium red onion, cut into quarters, layers separated (about 24 pieces)
>
> 1 large red bell pepper, seeded and cut into 24 large squares
>
> 1 large green bell pepper, seeded and cut into 24 large squares
>
> ½ medium eggplant, cut in 24 1-inch cubes
>
> 1 pound tempeh, cut into 24 1-inch cubes
>
> 2½ cups Orange Sauce (see sidebar)

1. Soak twelve 9-inch wooden skewers in water for half an hour. This will keep the skewers from burning.

2. Thread the vegetables and tempeh on the skewers in the following order: onion, red pepper, green pepper, eggplant, tempeh. Marinate the skewers in the orange sauce for 2 hours or up to 24 hours.

3. Prepare an outdoor grill or preheat the broiler. Grill skewers for 15 minutes, turning once or twice, until grill marks are visible. Serve hot.

SERVES 6 AS A MAIN COURSE, 12 AS A SIDE DISH

Calories	Total Protein	Soy Protein	Carbohydrate	Fat	Cholesterol	Fiber	Sodium
249	15 g	14 g	21 g	13 g	0 mg	0.7 g	78 mg

Information is for 2 kabobs.

Orange Sauce

2 cups orange juice
½ cup olive oil
6 garlic cloves, minced
1 large rosemary sprig, finely chopped
½ teaspoon salt
¼ teaspoon pepper

1. Combine all of the ingredients and stir well.
2. Refrigerate until ready to use. Sauce can be kept, refrigerated, for up to 2 weeks.

MAKES 2½ CUPS

Marinating

Marinades—such as Orange Sauce (page 155), Sweet and Sour Sauce (page 39), or Barbecue Sauce (page 154)—are a great way to add flavor to tempeh and tofu. Because these soy products, unlike meats, need no tenderizing, they don't require marinating more than an hour or two to be at their best. Tofu and tempeh are not as firm as meat, so marinate them in shallow pans and turn them gently to avoid breaking up the pieces. If you must marinate tofu or tempeh for a long period, limit the marinade to 24 hours, as the texture may break down, and be sure to store the marinating dish in the refrigerator to avoid spoilage.

Spinach Tempeh in Pastry Pockets

Enclosed in a golden crust, these spinach- and soy-filled bundles are cholesterol free, nutritious, and, thanks to ready-made puff pastry, easy to make. Garnish with broiled tomatoes and serve with a good red wine. Topped off with Peaches and Cream Brûlée (page 202), this makes a truly memorable meal.

3 10-ounce packages frozen chopped spinach, thawed
½ cup walnuts
6 scallions, white and tender green parts, sliced
6 garlic cloves, minced
2 teaspoons low-sodium soy sauce

1½ pounds firm tofu, crumbled
3 8-ounce packages tempeh
3 packages (1 pound, 1¼ ounces each) frozen puff pastry sheets, thawed for ½ hour
2 cups Espagnole Sauce (page 136)

1. Squeeze the spinach by handfuls to remove excess liquid.
2. Place the walnuts in a food processor or blender and process until they are finely ground.
3. In a large mixing bowl, combine the spinach, scallions, garlic, soy sauce, tofu, and walnuts. Set aside.
4. Preheat the oven to 400°F.
5. Cut each 8-ounce piece of tempeh into quarters. In a steamer basket set over boiling water, steam the tempeh pieces for 5 minutes.
6. Unfold the pastry onto a lightly floured surface and cut each sheet in half.
7. To assemble individual Pastry Pockets spread a puff pastry piece on a lightly floured surface and center a piece of tempeh on it. Top with ⅔ cup spinach-tofu filling. Top with another piece of tempeh and wrap the pastry dough around the layers. Fold the edges upward and pinch the dough tightly to seal. Turn the pastry over and place in baking pan seam side down, and bake for 20 minutes.
8. Warm the sauce in a small saucepan and spoon about ¼ cup onto each of 6 plates. Place a Pastry Pocket on top of the sauce and serve immediately.

SERVES 6

Calories	Total Protein	Soy Protein	Carbohydrate	Fat	Cholesterol	Fiber	Sodium
754	42.5 g	30 g	69.5 g	37.5 g	0 mg	12 g	653.5 mg

Information is for 1 pastry, including sauce.

Soy Sausage-Stuffed Cabbage Rolls

One internationally popular way of dressing up plain green cabbage is to stuff its leaves with a savory mixture and slow-cook it in a rich sauce. The fillings vary— you'll find sage and pork stuffed cabbage in France; ground beef or ham-stuffed cabbage in England; bulgur wheat and parsley-stuffed cabbage in the Middle East; and rice, olive, and pine nut-stuffed cabbage in Greece. In this recipe, tender cabbage leaves enclose a "meaty" filling of soy sausage and rice and garlic, all bathed in a flavorful tomato sauce. Serve this rib-sticking main course with Soy Caesar Salad with Herbed Croutons (page 53) and Soy Herb Bread (page 104).

1 large head green cabbage

4 bay leaves

6 garlic cloves, coarsely chopped

2 tablespoons vegetable oil

1 large onion, finely chopped

2 14-ounce packages beef-flavored
    soy sausage

1 cup rice

¼ teaspoon salt

2 teaspoons Worcestershire sauce

½ teaspoon white pepper

3 cups Tomato Sauce (page 111)

1. Select a large, shallow casserole with a tight cover and grease it lightly.

2. Carefully remove 12 large leaves from the cabbage and set aside. Shred enough of the remaining cabbage to make 1 cup; reserve the rest for another use. Put the shredded cabbage, bay leaves, and garlic in the bottom of the casserole.

3. In a separate pan, blanch the reserved cabbage leaves in boiling water for 3 minutes. Remove and set aside.

4. Heat the oil in a large skillet over high heat and sauté the onion and sausage for 3 minutes. Reduce the heat and add the rice, salt, Worcestershire sauce, and pepper. Mix well.

5. Divide the mixture among the 12 cabbage leaves, rolling each one up, tucking the ends toward the center and fastening with a toothpick. Place in the casserole dish. Pour the sauce over the rolls, cover, and simmer for 30 minutes.

SERVES 6

Calories	Total Protein	Soy Protein	Carbohydrate	Fat	Cholesterol	Fiber	Sodium
354	21 g	15 g	54 g	6 g	0 mg	9 g	755 mg

Information is for 2 stuffed cabbage leaves.

Mexican-Style Soy Sausage

A thick, hearty dish enlivened by the traditional south-of-the-border touch of unsweetened chocolate. Served with brown rice or warm corn tortillas, this makes a filling meal. Add a green salad with Creamy Garlic Dressing (page 54) and Tofu Flan (page 205) for a perfect Sunday night supper.

4 tablespoons olive oil

1 large onion, chopped

2 14-ounce packages beef-flavored
   soy sausage

2 garlic cloves, finely minced

5 ripe, medium tomatoes, chopped

1 tablespoon crushed red pepper

2 tablespoons chili powder

1 teaspoon ground cinnamon

1 teaspoon ground cumin

1 teaspoon salt, or to taste

⅓ cup unsweetened cocoa powder

2 cups Vegetable Stock, or as
   needed (page 120)

1. Heat the oil in a large saucepan over high heat and sauté the onion and sausage, stirring well, until browned, about 8 minutes. Add the garlic and sauté for 30 more seconds.

2. Lower the heat to medium-low. One at a time, add the tomatoes, red pepper, chili powder, cinnamon, and cumin, stirring well after each addition. Add salt to taste. Add the cocoa and mix well. Stir frequently as the mixture starts to thicken.

3. Simmer over very low heat for 1 hour, adding stock ½ cup at a time as needed to keep the mixture from getting too thick. Serve hot.

SERVES 6

Calories	Total Protein	Soy Protein	Carbohydrate	Fat	Cholesterol	Fiber	Sodium
228	17 g	16 g	24 g	7.7 g	0 mg	5 g	18.6 mg

Information is for a 1-cup serving.

Soy Hungarian Goulash

The original Hungarian goulash, a chunky beef stew infused with paprika, dates back almost a thousand years. This delicious up-to-date version uses soy sausage in place of the beef. Imported sweet paprika (available in the spice or gourmet section of grocery stores)—rather than the bland, domestic sort—makes all the difference. Goulash is usually enriched with sour cream, and you can add soy sour cream to the stew as it finishes cooking or pass around the table to dollop on top.

2 tablespoons vegetable oil

1 large onion, chopped

2 14-ounce packages beef-flavored
   soy sausage

6 garlic cloves, minced

2 tablespoons imported sweet
   paprika

3 cups Vegetable Stock (page 120)

½ cup dry white wine

2 cups strained sauerkraut

8 large button mushrooms,
   quartered

3 tablespoons caraway seeds

12 ounces flat noodles

1 cup soy sour cream (optional)

1. Heat the oil in a large saucepan over high heat and sauté the onion and sausage until the sausage browns, about 8 minutes. Stir frequently to prevent the soy sausage from sticking.

2. Add the garlic and paprika, stirring until the onion is well coated with paprika, about 1 minute.

3. Add the stock, wine, sauerkraut, mushrooms, and caraway seeds. Reduce the heat and simmer for 30 minutes.

4. While the goulash is simmering, cook the noodles. Set aside and keep warm.

5. If you are using the sour cream, add it to the goulash by spoonfuls, stirring after each addition, and simmer for 5 minutes. Do not bring to a boil. (Alternatively, omit the sour cream here and serve it on the side at the table.)

6. Spoon the goulash over the hot noodles and serve immediately.

SERVES 6

Calories	Total Protein	Soy Protein	Carbohydrate	Fat	Cholesterol	Fiber	Sodium
455	26 g	16 g	71 g	6.5 g	0 mg	8 g	1069 mg

Information is per serving.

Soy Meat Loaf

The reason your mother made meat loaf, and her mother made meat loaf, and her mother's mother made meat loaf, is that it is an incredibly quick, easy, inexpensive, and satisfying meal. We may make fun of it, but meat loaf is a comfort food that will always be around. This version uses soy sausage instead of ground beef or turkey, with plenty of spices for zest. Serve with Garlic Mashed Potatoes with Soy Milk (page 55) and Creamed Spinach (page 65).

3 14-ounce packages beef-flavored
  soy sausage
2½ cups plain bread crumbs,
  packaged or homemade
1 large carrot, chopped
1 medium onion, chopped
6 garlic cloves, minced

2 teaspoons dried basil
2 teaspoons dried thyme
2 teaspoons dried oregano
2 teaspoons dried tarragon
1 teaspoon black pepper
1½ cups tomato paste
1 cup Tomato Sauce (page 111)

1. Preheat the oven to 350° F. and lightly grease a medium baking pan.
2. Crumble the soy sausage in a large mixing bowl. Add the bread crumbs, carrot, onion, garlic, basil, thyme, oregano, tarragon, and pepper, mixing thoroughly.
3. Stir in the tomato paste thoroughly. Shape the mixture into 2 small loaves and place in the baking pan.
4. Bake the loaves for 30 minutes, until loaf browns slightly. Brush the top of each loaf with the sauce, and bake for 5 more minutes.
5. Meanwhile, heat the remaining tomato sauce in a separate pan. Remove meat loaves from oven, slice, and serve hot. Pass the warmed tomato sauce on the side.

SERVES 6

Calories	Total Protein	Soy Protein	Carbohydrate	Fat	Cholesterol	Fiber	Sodium
364	24 g	16 g	51 g	3 g	0 mg	8 g	908.5 mg

Information is for ⅓ of a loaf, including sauce.

Polenta with Mushroom and Soy Sausage Ragout

Anything you can do with pasta, you can do with polenta, an Italian cornmeal mush that has become increasingly popular in restaurant and home kitchens alike. This recipe uses polenta as the bed for a savory mushroom-soy sausage ragout. It can be made with either ready-made polenta or homemade.

½ cup olive oil
24 small Italian-style soy sausage
   links, cut into large slices
2 medium onions, finely chopped
4 large white mushrooms, finely
   chopped
1½ teaspoons crushed dried
   rosemary

1 teaspoon Italian seasoning
1¼ cups dry white wine
Salt and pepper to taste
2 14-ounce packages ready-made
   polenta, available in refrigerated
   section of market, or Soy Polenta
   (page 184)

1. In a large, heavy skillet, heat ¼ cup of the olive oil and sauté the sausage until well browned, about 5 minutes. Remove the sausage and set aside.

2. In the same skillet, heat the remaining ¼ cup olive oil. Add the onions, mushrooms, rosemary, and Italian seasoning, sautéing until browned, about 8 minutes. Lower the heat and return the sausage to the pan.

3. Stir in the wine, cover the pot, and cook for 5 minutes. Season with salt and pepper. Set lid askew and simmer for 20 more minutes.

4. While the sausage is simmering, preheat the oven to 350°F. Slice the ready-made polenta into 18 pieces and place on parchment-lined baking sheets. (If using homemade polenta, follow instructions in the recipe.) Bake for 20 minutes, turning once, at 10 minutes.

5. Arrange 3 slices on each of 6 plates and spoon about 1 cup of sausage mixture over it. Serve immediately.

SERVES 6

Calories	Total Protein	Soy Protein	Carbohydrate	Fat	Cholesterol	Fiber	Sodium
705	30 g	21 g	58 g	36 g	0 mg	0 g	864 mg

Information is for 3 slices of polenta, including 1 cup ragout.

Soy Sausage Paella

This traditional Spanish dish takes its name from the open pan in which it is cooked. Paellas differ radically—some include lobster and mussels, some chicken and duck, some artichokes and peas—but they all start out with rice, olive oil, garlic, and saffron. This version contains these paella essentials and also incorporates soy sausage. Experiment by adding other vegetables, such as peas or asparagus tips. Experimentation is what paella is all about.

1 tablespoon olive oil, or more as needed	½ teaspoon saffron threads
1 14-ounce package ground soy sausage	1½ cups arborio rice
1 medium red onion, chopped	4 cups Vegetable Stock (page 120)
½ large red bell pepper, seeded and chopped	1 14-ounce can soybeans, drained
2 garlic cloves, minced	1 14-ounce can artichoke hearts, drained and quartered
1½ cups tomato puree	½ teaspoon black pepper
1 teaspoon crushed, dried rosemary	⅓ cup chopped parsley
	Soy parmesan cheese, to taste (optional)

1. In a paella pan or large skillet, heat the oil over medium heat and cook the sausage, stirring frequently, for about 5 minutes, or until brown. Do not break the sausage chunks up too finely, as the dish should have a meaty texture. Remove from the pan and set aside.

2. In the same pan, sauté the onion and bell pepper over medium-high heat until brown, 5 to 8 minutes. Add the garlic and cook for another 30 seconds.

3. Add the cooked sausage, the tomato puree, and rosemary, and cook until the mixture thickens slightly, about 10 minutes.

4. Add the saffron and rice, stirring thoroughly. Add the stock, ½-cup at a time, stirring constantly, until the liquid is absorbed before adding more stock. This process takes about 30 minutes. If the mixture gets too dry, add more stock.

5. Add the soybeans, artichoke hearts, pepper, and parsley, stirring to combine. Cook for another 5 minutes. Serve immediately, topped with soy parmesan cheese, if desired.

SERVES 6

Calories	Total Protein	Soy Protein	Carbohydrate	Fat	Cholesterol	Fiber	Sodium
508	30 g	22 g	85 g	11 g	0 mg	10 g	511 mg

Information is for a 2-cup serving.

Sautéed Spinach and Garlic Tempeh

This is a dish I created in a pinch for unexpected dinner guests, using only the ingredients I had on hand at the time. It was a hit: the soy sauce and garlic lend an Asian flavor to this delicious stir-fry. I served it over rice that night, but I have since used the mixture as a topping for pasta or polenta.

1 tablespoon vegetable oil
½ small onion, chopped
6 garlic cloves, minced
¼ cup low-sodium soy sauce
2 pounds tempeh, chopped
2 10-ounce packages frozen chopped spinach,
     thawed and drained
Salt and pepper to taste

1. Heat the oil in a medium pan over high heat and sauté the onion for 5 minutes. Add the garlic and cook for 30 seconds more.
2. Add the soy sauce and tempeh, and reduce the heat to low. Let the mixture simmer for 5 minutes, stirring occasionally. Add the spinach and cook until spinach is heated through, about 5 minutes. Add salt and pepper to taste.
3. Serve hot.

SERVES 6

Calories	Total Protein	Soy Protein	Carbohydrate	Fat	Cholesterol	Fiber	Sodium
505	36 g	28 g	63 g	15 g	0 mg	10 g	497 mg

Information is for a 1-cup serving.

Cajun Red Hot Jambalaya
with Soy Sausage

As spirited as the New Orleans original, this favorite Cajun dish incorporates soy sausage for heartiness without cholesterol and saturated fat. The heat comes from the cayenne pepper, which can easily be adjusted to individual taste. Feel free to substitute brown rice for white, if desired, but add 30 minutes to the overall cooking time. This recipe is easy to double or triple, and has therefore always been a sure-fire success when feeding large groups. Serve it with Soy Herb Bread (page 104) and a salad.

1 tablespoon vegetable oil

1 10-ounce package lean soy
   sausage links, sliced

2 large onions, chopped (about
   2 cups)

3 celery stalks, chopped (about
   1 cup)

1 large green pepper, seeded and
   chopped (about 1 cup)

3 small bay leaves, crushed

6 garlic cloves, chopped

2 tablespoons Cajun seasoning

½ teaspoon salt

2 cups long-grain rice

3 cups tomato juice

3 cups Vegetable Stock (page 120)

1 pound ripe tomatoes, chopped, or
   1 14-ounce can chopped
   tomatoes, with juice

1 bunch scallions, chopped (about
   1 cup), green and white parts

1. In a large soup pot, heat the oil over medium-high heat and sauté the sausage slices for 5 minutes or until they are browned.

2. Add the onions, celery, green pepper, bay leaves, garlic, Cajun seasoning, and salt. Continue to cook for 10 to 12 minutes, stirring frequently, until the onions brown.

3. Stir in the rice and cook for 5 more minutes, stirring occasionally.

4. Add the tomato juice and stock, stirring well, and bring to a boil. Reduce the heat to medium and simmer, covered, for 15 minutes.

5. Add the tomatoes and scallions, stirring well.

6. Continue cooking over low heat, covered, until rice is tender, about 45 minutes. Serve hot.

SERVES 6

Calories	Total Protein	Soy Protein	Carbohydrate	Fat	Cholesterol	Fiber	Sodium
323	22 g	21 g	32 g	13 g	0 mg	3.5 g	219 mg

Information is for a 2-cup serving.

Arroz con Tempeh

This is a tempeh knockoff of arroz con pollo, *the famous saffron-infused Spanish dish of chicken* (pollo) *with onions, peppers, and rice* (arroz). *It works as an easy main course, with a green salad, or in combination with a vegetable dish such as Asparagus Spears with Garlic Aïoli (page 74).*

2 tablespoons olive oil

2 pounds tempeh, cut into strips

1 large onion, chopped

1 small green bell pepper, seeded and chopped

1 small red bell pepper, seeded and chopped

2 garlic cloves, minced

4 cups Vegetable Stock (page 120)

¼ teaspoon saffron threads

½ teaspoon cayenne pepper

2 cups long-grain rice

1 10-ounce package frozen peas

Salt and pepper to taste

1. Heat the oil in a large saucepan over high heat and sauté the tempeh, onions, and bell peppers until the tempeh is slightly browned, about 8 minutes. Add the garlic and cook for 1 more minute.

2. Add the stock, saffron, and cayenne, mixing well. Bring the mixture to a boil and stir in the rice. Reduce the heat to low, cover, and cook for 20 minutes. Stir in the peas and cook 5 minutes more, until the peas are thoroughly heated. Add salt and pepper to taste. Serve immediately.

SERVES 6

Calories	Total Protein	Soy Protein	Carbohydrate	Fat	Cholesterol	Fiber	Sodium
663	37 g	28 g	93 g	18 g	0 mg	9 g	39 mg

Information is for a 1½-cup serving.

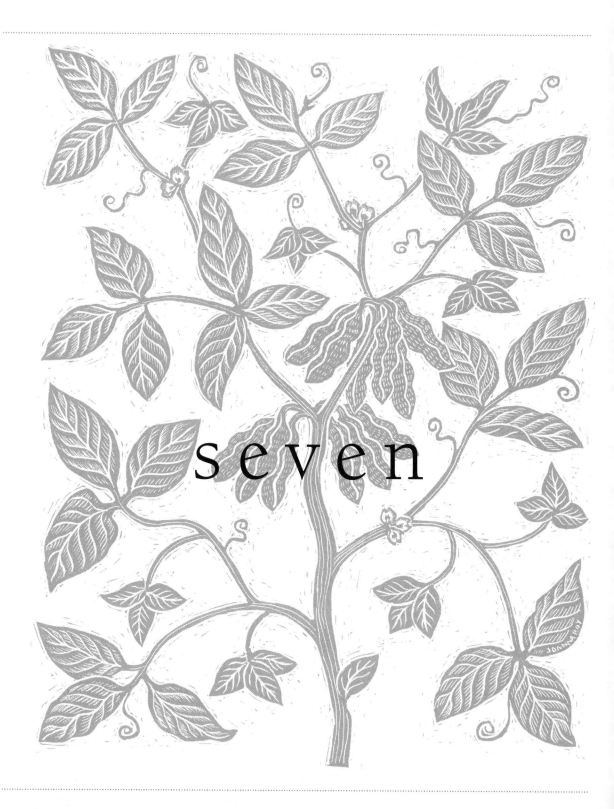

seven

pastas and grains

As Americans have become more and more health conscious, the emphasis in our diet has shifted from meat to grains. Pasta has therefore taken center stage as one of the most popular foods in the country, and with good reason. Beloved by adults and kids alike, it comes in all shapes and sizes, from basic spaghetti and macaroni to imported rotini and orrechiette. It can be stuffed with cheese, meat, or vegetables; topped with sauces ranging from simple tomato to hearty meat to piquant herb. Pasta can be homey and comforting, like macaroni and cheese, or thrilling and exotic, like Soy Tortellini with Carrot-Ginger Sauce.

Even better, it's the perfect backdrop for delicious and healthful soy-based sauces. Soy Fettuccine Alfredo, for example, features flat noodles in a luscious, creamy sauce made from soy milk and soy mozzarella. Based on the dish that is classically laden with heavy cream and butter, this healthful soy version has plenty of flavor, lush texture, lots of soy protein, but no cholesterol and remarkably little fat. Penne with Soy Sausage Bolognese uses soy "meat" instead of ground beef to create a hearty red sauce that brings out the best in any pasta, from spaghetti to penne to lasagna. The pasta dishes in these pages use a range of soy products: tofu, soy meats, soy milk, and soy cheese. I've also included recipes using delicious store-bought soy-filled tortellini and ravioli. These are widely available in health food stores and they freeze well, so it's easy to keep them on hand. Though you can use regular cheese-filled pastas in a pinch, using soy-filled pasta—in Soy Ravioli with Four Cheeses, for example—makes the dish especially satisfying as a main course, and dramatically increases the level of health-giving soy protein.

Other grains marry beautifully with soy, too. For example, sesame-scented Tempeh Fried Rice takes its inspiration from Chinese cooking, where rice and soy foods have long been deliciously paired.

Combining pastas and grains with soy can be as simple as sprinkling a few tablespoons of soy parmesan cheese on a bowl of hot risotto, or as detailed as layering soy cheeses and soy-based sauce in an appetizing lasagne. The recipes in this chapter will work equally well as main courses or in smaller portions as side dishes. However you choose to do it, combining soy with grains makes pastas and grains even easier to love.

Soy Fettuccine Alfredo

If you like fettuccine alfredo—that sinfully delicious combination of a cheese and cream sauce over flat noodles—you'll love this healthful version. It's every bit as luscious as the original, but contains no cholesterol, little fat, and all the benefits of 8 grams of soy protein.

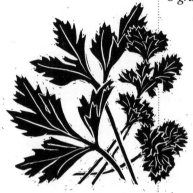

1 pound fettuccine noodles
1 tablespoon olive oil
6 garlic cloves, minced
2 cups low-fat soy milk
6 ounces soy mozzarella cheese, grated
¼ cup soy parmesan cheese
⅓ cup chopped parsley
Salt and white pepper to taste

1. Cook the pasta in plenty of boiling water until just al dente, and drain.
2. Heat the oil in a large pot over medium heat and sauté the garlic for a few minutes, without letting it brown. Stir in the soy milk.
3. Add the noodles, stirring to coat them with sauce and to prevent sticking.
4. Add the soy mozzarella and soy parmesan, stirring until the cheese melts and the sauce thickens.
5. Stir in the parsley, salt, and white pepper and serve immediately.

SERVES 6

Calories	Total Protein	Soy Protein	Carbohydrate	Fat	Cholesterol	Fiber	Sodium
334	17 g	8 g	47 g	8.7 g	0 mg	0 g	247 mg

Information is per serving.

Fusilli with Soy Pesto

Curly fusilli is the perfect pasta shape to capture this heavenly—and healthful—soy version of pesto. Soy parmesan cheese replaces its dairy counterpart here, reducing the fat and eliminating the cholesterol without affecting taste or texture in the slightest. In summer, when fresh basil is plentiful, I always make extra sauce to freeze. This recipe for pesto can be easily doubled and frozen in half-cup portions for later use.

1 pound fusilli pasta
2 cups basil leaves, chopped
3 garlic cloves
2 tablespoons pine nuts
½ cup soy parmesan cheese
¼ cup olive oil

1. Cook the fusilli in a large quantity of boiling water until al dente.
2. Meanwhile, put the basil, garlic, pine nuts, and soy parmesan cheese in a food processor or blender. Turn the blender or processor on medium speed and while it is running, drizzle in the olive oil until all ingredients are thoroughly combined.
3. Drain the fusilli and pour the pesto over it. Toss lightly to combine. Serve warm or at room temperature.

SERVES 6

Calories	Total Protein	Soy Protein	Carbohydrate	Fat	Cholesterol	Fiber	Sodium
345	16 g	6 g	53 g	9 g	0 mg	3.3 g	10 mg

Information is per serving.

Soy Ravioli with
Sun-Dried Tomato Cream Sauce

Delicious soy cheese–filled ravioli and tortellini are available in health food stores and some large markets. This creamy, rich sauce, which is studded with tangy sun-dried tomatoes, also tastes great on any plain pasta.

2 15-ounce packages soy ravioli

2 tablespoons olive oil

1 small onion, chopped

1 medium carrot, chopped

1 celery stalk, chopped

3 garlic cloves, minced

½ cup chopped sun-dried tomatoes in olive oil

2 teaspoons Italian seasoning

2 cups low-fat soy milk

¼ teaspoon salt

1. Cook the ravioli according to package directions.

2. Meanwhile, in a saucepan, heat the oil over high heat and sauté the onion, carrot, and celery for 3 minutes. Add the garlic and cook for 1 more minute.

3. Lower the heat to medium and add the sun-dried tomatoes and Italian seasoning, mixing well. Add the soy milk and salt and cook for 3 more minutes, until heated through.

4. Transfer to a food processor or blender and blend until smooth. Serve immediately over hot ravioli.

SERVES 6

Calories	Total Protein	Soy Protein	Carbohydrate	Fat	Cholesterol	Fiber	Sodium
415	13 g	10 g	62 g	11 g	0 mg	1 g	555 mg
95	3 g	2 g	8 g	6 g	0 mg	1 g	115 mg

Top row information is for 1 cup ravioli and ⅓ cup sauce. Bottom row information is for ⅓ cup sauce.

Soy Ravioli with Four Cheeses

A double delight for cheese lovers, this dish combines cheese-filled ravioli with a creamy, cheesy sauce. Though it sounds sinfully rich, it is free of cholesterol and provides a whopping 29 grams of soy protein. Look for soy ravioli in health food stores or larger markets, or try the sauce over elbow noodles for a delicious soy version of macaroni and cheese.

2 15-ounce packages soy ravioli

3 tablespoons soy margarine

1 cup soy milk

8 ounces soy cheddar cheese, finely grated

8 ounces garlic-and-herb soy mozzarella cheese, finely grated

8 ounces soy cream cheese

1½ cups soy parmesan cheese

Chopped parsley, for garnish

1. Prepare the ravioli according to package directions.

2. While the ravioli is cooking, heat the soy margarine and soy milk in a large saucepan over medium heat, stirring constantly with a wire whisk until the margarine is completely melted, about 2 minutes.

3. Lower the heat and add the cheeses one at a time, stirring until the sauce is smooth, about 10 minutes.

4. As the ravioli finishes cooking, drain it and place in a warm serving dish. Pour the cheese sauce over the ravioli, sprinkle with the parsley, and serve at once.

SERVES 6

Calories	Total Protein	Soy Protein	Carbohydrate	Fat	Cholesterol	Fiber	Sodium
607	30 g	29 g	57 g	23 g	0 mg	2 g	1025 mg
287	20 g	19 g	3 g	18 g	0 mg	0 g	585 mg

Top row information is for 1 cup ravioli and ¾ cup sauce. Bottom row information is for ¾ cup sauce.

Soy Tortellini with Carrot-Ginger Sauce

Hearty soy-cheese filled tortellini are perfectly balanced by a delicate sauce with the zing of fresh ginger. The slightly sweet sauce, a lovely pale orange puree of sautéed carrots and carrot juice, gets its tangy richness from the soy sour cream whisked in at the end. Serve Mixed Baby Greens with Mustard Tarragon Soy Vinaigrette (page 50) alongside.

1 tablespoon vegetable oil	1 cup carrot juice
1 medium onion, chopped	2 15-ounce packages soy tortellini
2 large carrots, chopped	1 cup soy sour cream
6 garlic cloves, coarsely chopped	1 teaspoon salt
1½-inch piece fresh ginger, minced	½ teaspoon white pepper

1. In a large saucepan, heat the oil over medium-high heat and sauté the onion and carrots, about 3 minutes. Lower the heat, add the garlic and ginger, and cook for 1 more minute.

2. Add the carrot juice and simmer for 20 minutes.

3. While the sauce is simmering, prepare the tortellini according to package directions and set aside.

4. Remove the sauce from the heat and puree in a food processor or blender.

5. Return the sauce to the pan and whisk in the soy sour cream, salt, and pepper. Simmer for 10 minutes or until the mixture is heated through. Pour over the hot tortellini and serve immediately.

SERVES 6

Calories	Total Protein	Soy Protein	Carbohydrate	Fat	Cholesterol	Fiber	Sodium
393	12 g	11 g	61 g	8 g	0 mg	4 g	848 mg
112	2 g	1 g	10 g	7 g	0 mg	2.6 g	397 mg

Top row information is for 1 cup tortellini and ⅓ cup sauce. Bottom row information is for ⅓ cup sauce.

Soy Cheese Manicotti

This is one of my favorite meals to serve dinner guests. Stuffed manicotti look impressive but are deceptively easy to prepare. You'd never guess this rich and cheesy version is filled with healthful soy cheese and tofu instead of the usual egg and ricotta combination. You can make these a day ahead and bake them at the last minute. For a heartier meal, blanket the manicotti with Soy Bolognese Sauce (page 176) instead of plain tomato sauce.

1 pound manicotti shells (2 boxes)

1½ pounds firm tofu

1 pound soy mozzarella cheese, shredded

1 cup soy parmesan cheese

¼ cup chopped Italian parsley

6 fresh basil leaves, chopped

1 sprig of oregano, chopped

½ teaspoon salt

½ teaspoon black pepper

4 cups Tomato Sauce, pureed (page 111)

1. Preheat the oven to 350°F. Lightly grease a 9 × 13-inch baking pan.

2. Cook the manicotti according to package directions, drain, and allow them to cool, making sure they are not sticking together.

3. In a large bowl, crumble the tofu and combine with three-fourths of the soy mozzarella, half of the soy parmesan, the parsley, basil, oregano, salt, and pepper. Mix thoroughly.

4. Carefully spoon about ⅓ cup of the mixture into each shell. Arrange in a single layer in the baking dish and cover with the tomato sauce. Sprinkle the remaining soy mozzarella and soy parmesan cheese on top and bake for 35 minutes, until cheese is bubbling.

SERVES 6 TO 8

Calories	Total Protein	Soy Protein	Carbohydrate	Fat	Cholesterol	Fiber	Sodium
479	33 g	18 g	46 g	17 g	0 mg	2 g	247 mg

Information is for 3 stuffed manicotti.

Tofu Lasagne

If you thought nothing could improve upon basic lasagne—those hearty layers of broad noodles encasing cheese, vegetables, herbs, and tomato sauce—think again. In this dish, you'll never notice that healthful crumbled tofu takes the place of the usual ricotta cheese, and soy mozzarella and soy parmesan replace their dairy counterparts. This Northern Italian–style lasagne gains richness from creamy Béchamel Sauce; if you'd like a "meaty" dish, substitute Soy Sausage Bolognese (page 176) for the tomato sauce. (And yes, you really do use uncooked noodles here; I promise they'll be done when you take the lasagne out of the oven.)

1½ pounds soft tofu, crumbled

10 large white mushrooms, chopped

1 teaspoon dried oregano

1 teaspoon dried basil

1 teaspoon dried thyme

3 cups Tomato Sauce, pureed (page 111)

½ pound lasagna noodles

2½ cups Béchamel Sauce (page 75)

8 ounces soy mozzarella cheese, shredded

¼ cup soy parmesan cheese

¼ cup water

1. Preheat the oven to 350°F. Lightly grease a 9 × 13-inch baking pan.

2. In a medium mixing bowl, thoroughly combine the tofu, mushrooms, oregano, basil, and thyme.

3. Spread about ½ cup of tomato sauce on the bottom of the baking pan. Top with a layer of uncooked lasagna noodles. Cover with another ½ cup of tomato sauce.

4. Evenly spread half of the tofu mixture over the noodles and cover with 1 cup of Béchamel Sauce. Cover with half of the shredded mozzarella. Top with another layer of noodles and about ½ cup of tomato sauce.

5. Spread the remaining tofu mixture over the noodles, layer on the béchamel and remaining mozzarella, and top that with a layer of noodles. Cover the top with about 1 cup of the tomato sauce and the parmesan.

6. Pour the water into the corner of the pan and cover pan with aluminum foil. Bake for 45 minutes, until mixture is bubbling. Let cool for 5 minutes before serving.

SERVES 6

Calories	Total Protein	Soy Protein	Carbohydrate	Fat	Cholesterol	Fiber	Sodium
166	17 g	9 g	20 g	11 g	0 mg	2.6 g	228 mg

Information is for a 4½ × 3½-inch piece.

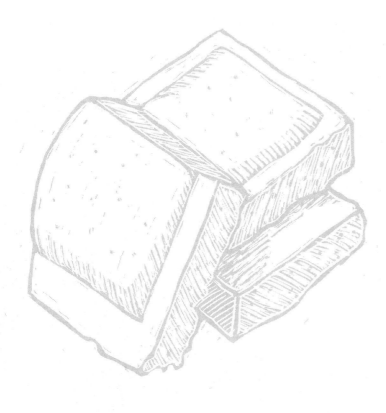

Penne with Soy Sausage Bolognese

In this version of a classic pasta dish from Northern Italy, soy sausage takes the place of the usual ground beef and tubular penne stands in for the traditional spaghetti. I think the result—a chunky, "meaty" red sauce that clings deliciously to the hollow pasta—is even more satisfying than the original. Serve with a green salad and Italian bread.

> 3 tablespoons olive oil
>
> 1 small onion, chopped
>
> 2 14-ounce packages ground soy sausage
>
> 2 garlic cloves, minced
>
> ½ cup dry red wine
>
> 10 plum tomatoes, coarsely chopped
>
> 1 tablespoon brown sugar
>
> ¼ cup chopped Italian parsley
>
> 1 pound penne pasta
>
> Soy parmesan cheese, for topping (optional)

1. Heat the oil in a large saucepan over high heat and sauté the onion and sausage until they are browned, about 8 minutes. Add the garlic and sauté for 30 more seconds.

2. Stir in the wine, tomatoes, brown sugar, and parsley. Lower the heat and simmer for 30 minutes.

3. Meanwhile, cook the pasta until al dente. Drain.

4. Toss pasta with sauce. Top with soy parmesan, if desired.

SERVES 6

Calories	Total Protein	Soy Protein	Carbohydrate	Fat	Cholesterol	Fiber	Sodium
202	20 g	16 g	17 g	6 g	0 mg	2 g	53 mg

Information is for 1⅓-cup serving, not including cheese.

Sunday Night Tofu Noodle Casserole

This casserole resembles a lasagne with its layers of cheese, noodles, and hearty sauce. It makes a great family supper. I often double this recipe and freeze one, tightly covered, for future use.

2 cups flat noodles

2 tablespoons vegetable oil

1 14-ounce package beef-flavored
   soy sausage

½ small onion, minced

½ small green bell pepper, seeded
   and chopped

2 cups Tomato Sauce (page 111)

1 teaspoon Worcestershire sauce

12 ounces firm tofu, crumbled

6 ounces soy cream cheese

⅓ cup soy sour cream

1 tablespoon chopped chives

½ teaspoon salt

1. Cook noodles until just al dente and set aside.

2. Preheat the oven to 350°F. and lightly grease a 2-quart casserole dish.

3. Heat the oil in a skillet over medium heat and sauté the soy sausage, onion, and green pepper until sausage is slightly browned, about 5 minutes. Add the tomato sauce and Worcestershire sauce. Reduce the heat to low and simmer for 5 minutes. Remove from the heat and set aside.

4. In a medium bowl, thoroughly combine the crumbled tofu, soy cream cheese, soy sour cream, chives, and salt.

5. Spread a small amount of soy sausage sauce evenly over the bottom of the casserole and top with half of the noodles. Cover with the cheese mixture, then the remaining noodles and soy sausage sauce.

6. Bake for 50 minutes or until bubbling. Serve hot.

SERVES 6

Calories	Total Protein	Soy Protein	Carbohydrate	Fat	Cholesterol	Fiber	Sodium
510	19 g	19 g	73 g	19 g	0 mg	3.5 g	750 mg

Information is per serving.

Soba Noodles with
Spicy Tofu Peanut Sauce

To my mind, this dish is one of the reasons Chinese restaurants exist. Ginger, garlic, and cayenne pepper combine with peanut butter to make an incredibly delicious, velvety sauce that's the perfect foil for soft buckwheat soba noodles. A friend of mine once bet that I couldn't come up with a soy version as satisfying as the original. This recipe proved him wrong. The classic version of this dish calls for a lot of oil; I've replaced it with soy milk and pureed tofu, which make the dish creamier as well as healthier. Serve hot, cold, or at room temperature.

2 pounds soba noodles (available in large grocery stores, health food stores, or Asian markets)

Spicy Tofu Peanut Sauce

6 tablespoons minced cilantro

2 large cucumbers, peeled, seeded, and sliced into matchsticks

2 bunches chopped scallions (about 2 cups), green and white parts

12 ounces firm tofu

2 garlic cloves, minced

1 1-inch piece fresh ginger, minced

½ tablespoon cayenne pepper

¼ cup soy sauce

2 tablespoons honey

½ cup soy milk

1 cup natural chunky peanut butter

1. Have all ingredients, especially peanut butter and honey, at room temperature before preparing recipe.

2. Cook the pasta according to the package directions, drain, and cool to room temperature.

3. Transfer the noodles to a large bowl. Add the cilantro and cucumbers and 5 tablespoons of scallions to the noodles. Toss gently and set aside.

4. In a food processor or blender, whip the tofu until smooth. Add the garlic, ginger, cayenne, and soy sauce and process or blend briefly until combined.

5. In a medium saucepan, over moderate heat, combine the honey, soy milk, and peanut butter and stir constantly until mixed.

6. Remove from heat and add the tofu mixture, beating vigorously with a wire whip.

7. Divide the soba noodles evenly among 6 serving plates. Spoon the sauce over the noodles and garnish with reserved scallions.

SERVES 6

Calories	Total Protein	Soy Protein	Carbohydrate	Fat	Cholesterol	Fiber	Sodium
559	26 g	5 g	98 g	12 g	0 mg	6 g	1250 mg

Information is for a 2-cup serving.

Orange Soy-Nut Brown Rice

Creamy with soy sour cream and studded with crunchy soy nuts and flecks of orange zest, this hearty rice dish has an autumnal feel. A slightly sweet dish, this glorified rice goes best with simple entrees such as Broiled Tofu with Five-Onion Sauce (page 143).

2 cups orange juice
2 cups Vegetable Stock (page 120)
2 cups brown rice

1 cup soy sour cream
½ cup chopped soy nuts
Zest of 1 orange

1. Bring the orange juice and stock to a boil. Add the rice and bring to a second boil. Reduce the heat, cover, and simmer for 40 minutes. The rice should be very tender and all the water absorbed.

2. When the rice is fully cooked, stir in the soy sour cream until heated thoroughly, and fold in the soy nuts and orange zest. Serve immediately.

SERVES 6

Calories	Total Protein	Soy Protein	Carbohydrate	Fat	Cholesterol	Fiber	Sodium
386	10 g	4 g	64 g	5 g	0 mg	3.5 g	141 mg

Information is per serving.

Tempeh Fried Rice

Chinese fried rice is typically a catch-all for whatever leftovers you have in the refrigerator. It usually contains a variety of vegetables like peas and scallions, along with pork, chicken, shrimp, or egg strips, mixed into white rice and stir-fried in hot oil. This version replaces the meat with tempeh and omits the egg, but none of the flavor. Serve with Garden Kabobs with Orange Sauce (page 155).

3 tablespoons vegetable oil

3 tablespoons toasted sesame oil

2 tablespoons low-sodium soy sauce

1 pound tempeh, crumbled

3 garlic cloves, minced

6 scallions, thinly sliced, green and white parts

1 cup frozen peas, rinsed in warm water and drained

1 cup canned water chestnuts, drained and thinly sliced

4 cups cooked rice

1 teaspoon crushed red pepper

½ teaspoon salt

1. In a large sauté pan or wok, heat the vegetable oil, sesame oil, and soy sauce over high heat. Add the tempeh and sauté for 3 minutes.

2. Add the garlic, scallions, peas, and water chestnuts, and continue to sauté for another minute.

3. Add the rice and mix thoroughly until all the ingredients are combined. Sauté rice for another 3 minutes, constantly stirring.

4. Stir in the crushed red pepper and salt and serve immediately.

SERVES 6

Calories	Total Protein	Soy Protein	Carbohydrate	Fat	Cholesterol	Fiber	Sodium
365	14 g	12 g	45 g	14 g	0 mg	4.5 g	337 mg

Information is for a 1½-cup serving.

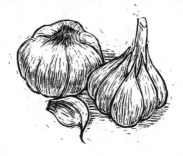

Soy Parmesan Risotto

Short, plump arborio rice (available in most grocery stores) absorbs flavorful stock and seasonings while it simmers, resulting in a creamy Italian specialty. You have to stir the rice while it slowly cooks, but it's well worth the effort. Vary this recipe, if you wish, by stirring in small quantities of peas, asparagus tips, or cooked soy bacon or sausage. Accompanied by a green salad, risotto can make a deliciously simple meal on its own, or serve it with Tofu Cacciatore (page 142).

3 tablespoons olive oil
1 small onion, finely chopped
2 cups arborio rice
1 teaspoon saffron threads
6 cups Vegetable Stock (page 120), heated
½ cup soy parmesan cheese
Salt and white pepper to taste

1. Heat the olive oil in a large saucepan over medium heat and sauté the onion for 5 minutes. Add the rice and stir to coat, sautéing for about 1 minute more so that rice browns slightly.

2. Reduce the heat and add the saffron and ½ cup of the stock, stirring constantly until all the liquid is absorbed. Continue to add stock, ½ cup at a time, stirring until all the liquid is absorbed and the rice is tender. This takes about 25 minutes.

3. Gently stir in the soy parmesan cheese and salt and pepper to taste. Serve immediately.

SERVES 6

Calories	Total Protein	Soy Protein	Carbohydrate	Fat	Cholesterol	Fiber	Sodium
364	7.5 g	2 g	62 g	9 g	0 mg	3 g	126 mg

Information is per serving.

Spanish Brown Rice Pilaf

Pilaf, which comes from the Persian word for rice, refers to any dish in which rice is sautéed in oil or butter before liquid is added. Pilafs are always enhanced by spices and seasonings and are usually cooked in flavorful stock rather than water. In this version, the flecks of green pepper and onion, along with rosy paprika, lend a Spanish feel. Serve with Tofu with Mexican Mole Sauce (page 140) or Tempeh Fajitas (page 152).

1½ tablespoons vegetable oil
½ medium onion, minced
½ small green bell pepper, minced
2 teaspoons paprika
2 cups brown rice
2 cups Vegetable Stock (page 120)
1½ cups soy milk

1. Heat the oil in a large saucepan over high heat and sauté the onion, green pepper, and paprika until the onion is translucent, 3 to 5 minutes. Add the rice and stir until it is completely coated with the mixture.
2. Add the stock and soy milk and bring to a boil. Reduce the heat to low and cook, covered, for 45 minutes, until rice is cooked.

SERVES 6

Calories	Total Protein	Soy Protein	Carbohydrate	Fat	Cholesterol	Fiber	Sodium
268	7 g	2 g	54 g	3.5 g	0 mg	6 g	24 mg

Information is for a 1-cup serving.

Soy Cheddar Pilaf

Another pilaf of sautéed rice and onions, this dish incorporates peas for colorful punctuation. Slivered almonds lend a crunchy texture to the chewy brown rice, and soy cheddar cheese adds richness, as well as soy protein. A perfect accompaniment to Broiled Tofu with Five-Onion Sauce (page 143), this pilaf also makes a great lunch—if there are any leftovers.

> 3 tablespoons vegetable oil
>
> 1 large onion, chopped
>
> 2 cups brown rice
>
> 4 cups Vegetable Stock (page 120)
>
> 1 teaspoon salt
>
> 1½ cups fresh or thawed frozen peas
>
> 1 cup almond slivers, toasted
>
> 8 ounces soy cheddar cheese, shredded

1. Heat the oil in a large saucepan over medium heat and sauté the onion until translucent, about 5 minutes. Add the rice and cook, stirring to coat with the oil, for 1 minute.

2. Add the stock and salt. Bring to a boil, reduce the heat to low, cover, and simmer for 40 minutes, until all the liquid is absorbed.

3. Quickly fold in the peas and almonds, cover, and cook for 10 more minutes.

4. Add the shredded cheese, stirring carefully so as not to break the grains. Serve immediately.

SERVES 6

Calories	Total Protein	Soy Protein	Carbohydrate	Fat	Cholesterol	Fiber	Sodium
573	19.5 g	8 g	68 g	26 g	0 mg	8 g	667 mg

Information is for a 1-cup serving.

Soy Polenta

Polenta is a traditional Italian side dish made with cornmeal. It can be served in different ways: soft like mush; or cooled, and sliced, then baked, fried, or grilled. You can top it with almost any pasta sauce, or with an entree that goes over noodles, such as Penne with Soy Sausage Bolognese (page 176) or Sautéed Spinach and Garlic Tempeh (page 163). While you can find ready-made polenta in many markets, it's so easy to make yourself. Use regular yellow cornmeal or polenta meal (a coarser grind of cornmeal). This version substitutes soy milk for the usual water, adding a substantial amount of healthful soy protein per serving.

> 6 cups soy milk
> ½ teaspoon salt
> 2 tablespoons soy margarine
> 2 cups yellow cornmeal or polenta meal

1. In a large saucepan, over high heat, combine the soy milk, salt, and margarine and bring to a boil.
2. Slowly add the cornmeal or polenta meal and reduce heat to low. Cook for 25 to 30 minutes, stirring frequently. The polenta will be soft. Ladle it onto a warm platter, cover with the chosen topping, and serve.

SERVES 6

Calories	Total Protein	Soy Protein	Carbohydrate	Fat	Cholesterol	Fiber	Sodium
202	10 g	6.6 g	35 g	7.3 g	0 mg	7.8 g	221 mg

Information is per serving.

Variation: When the polenta is ready, pour the mixture onto a parchment paper–lined cookie sheet and bake for 30 minutes at 350°F. Cut the polenta into 18 triangles and grill on a hot grill for 3 minutes on each side.

Couscous and Cranberries

Nothing could be simpler than this delicious rice alternative. Couscous is a traditional North African dish made from semolina. The grainlike pasta is steamed above a flavorful broth until tender and fluffy, and then served with meat or vegetable stews. Nowadays, instant couscous produces the same light results with absolutely no fuss. Inspired by Moroccan cooking, which often adds dried fruit to couscous dishes, I've added tart cranberries to perk up the mild-tasting grain. This is the perfect match for Near Eastern Curried Tempeh (page 151).

> 4 cups soy milk
> 4 cups instant couscous
> ¼ cup dried cranberries

1. In a large soup pot, bring the soy milk to a boil, and stir in the couscous.
2. Immediately remove from the stove and stir until all the soy milk is absorbed. Let sit 5 minutes.
3. Gently fold in the cranberries, and serve.

SERVES 6

Calories	Total Protein	Soy Protein	Carbohydrate	Fat	Cholesterol	Fiber	Sodium
519	20 g	4.5 g	99 g	4 g	0 mg	20 g	31 mg

Information is for a 1½-cup serving.

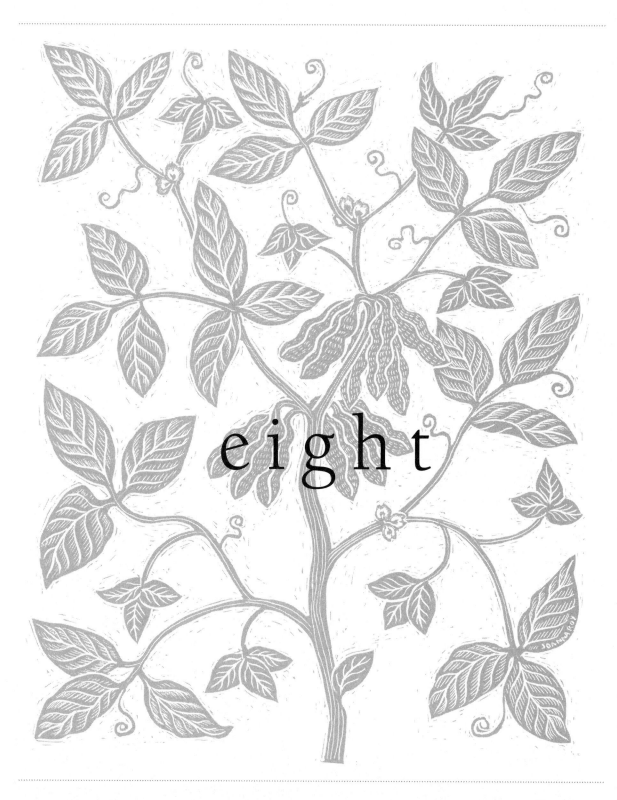

eight

desserts

The desserts in this chapter—from luscious Chocolate Almond Tofu Pie to yummy Chocolate Soy Brownies to the rich Yellow Cake with Chocolate Tofu Ganache—are sweets that truly combine good health with great taste. These recipes incorporate soy milk, soy cream cheese, soy yogurt, and tofu, among other soy foods. The results are desserts that taste for all the world as if they contained eggs, butter, and real dairy products. You won't believe that dense Tofu Cheesecake could taste so incredible and yet provide 5 grams of soy protein with absolutely no cholesterol. From homey Oatmeal Raisin Cookies to decadent Tofu Chocolate Mousse; spicy Tofu Pumpkin Pie to scrumptious Soy Tiramisù, there's a to-die-for treat to suit every taste.

Most of these desserts are amazingly simple to prepare. In contrast to traditional mousses and puddings, which require slowly cooked eggs and careful mixing to achieve a proper consistency, pureed tofu allows you to whip up luscious, creamy desserts with very little effort. Tofu substituted for eggs in the yellow cake make it as moist as a pudding cake, with a lot less fuss. Other soy ingredients function just as their dairy counterparts: soy cream cheese produces silky cheesecakes almost identical to the traditional favorite; the only difference is that, because of their low fat content, soy cheesecakes are cooked at a slightly lower temperature than those made with real cream cheese. Soy sour cream makes a tangy topping in Peaches and Cream Brûlée, and soy yogurt and soy milk add richness and moistness to Chocolate Soy Brownies. Tofu chocolate chips, in which tofu replaces some of the fat and all of the milk in ordinary chocolate, can be used in cookies and bars or melted just like regular chocolate chips. And they're just as hard to stop nibbling once you open the bag.

Try them all and see: these unbelievably delicious desserts will satisfy your sweet tooth as well as your conscience.

Chocolate Soy Brownies

Everyone loves brownies. This recipe, which incorporates soy milk and soy yogurt, produces cakelike rather than fudgy brownies. Adding a half-cup of walnuts or tofu chocolate chips makes these even more irresistible.

1½ cups unbleached all-purpose flour

2 teaspoons baking soda

1 cup sugar

½ cup unsweetened cocoa powder

4 ounces plain soy yogurt

1 cup nonfat soy milk

1 tablespoon vegetable oil

1 teaspoon vanilla extract

1. Preheat the oven to 425°F. and grease an 8×8-inch square pan or line with parchment paper.

2. In a large bowl, combine the flour, baking soda, sugar, and cocoa and set aside.

3. In a food processor or blender, mix the yogurt, soy milk, oil, and vanilla until smooth. Pour the yogurt mixture into the dry ingredients, stirring until well combined.

4. Pour the batter into the greased pan and bake for 25 minutes, or until the brownies spring back when touched.

5. Cool the brownies to room temperature before slicing.

MAKES 16

Calories	Total Protein	Soy Protein	Carbohydrate	Fat	Cholesterol	Fiber	Sodium
113	2.8 g	1.5 g	22 g	1.7 g	0 mg	0 g	110 mg

Information is for 1 brownie.

Oatmeal Raisin Cookies

As delicious as the ones in Grandma's cookie jar, but with a little soy goodness thrown in. These are guaranteed to disappear fast. Replace the raisins with the same amount of tofu chocolate chips (or regular chocolate chips) for a chewy, oatmeal-chocolate chip version.

1⅓ cups unbleached all-purpose
  flour
2 cups quick-cooking rolled oats
  (not instant)
½ teaspoon baking soda
¼ teaspoon salt
1 cup brown sugar

3 tablespoons soy margarine
1 cup soy milk
½ teaspoon vanilla extract
½ cup raisins or tofu chocolate
  chips (available in heath food
  stores)
¼ cup soy nuts

1. Preheat the oven to 350°F. and grease 2 cookie sheets lightly or line them with parchment paper.

2. In a large mixing bowl, combine the flour, oats, baking soda, and salt.

3. In a medium bowl, beat the brown sugar and soy margarine with an electric mixer until creamy. Add the soy milk and vanilla, mixing thoroughly.

4. Gradually add the liquid mixture to the flour and oats and stir by hand until well combined. Fold in the raisins or chocolate chips and the soy nuts.

5. Drop the dough by tablespoonfuls onto the cookie sheets. Space the cookies about 2 inches apart.

6. Bake for 15 to 18 minutes or until light golden brown. Allow to cool slightly before removing from cookie sheets.

MAKES 32 COOKIES

Calories	Total Protein	Soy Protein	Carbohydrate	Fat	Cholesterol	Fiber	Sodium
76	1.5 g	0.5 g	14 g	1.6 g	14 mg	0.5 g	33 mg

Information is for 1 cookie.

Black and White Soy Cookies

These impressive-looking checkerboard cookies, combining vanilla and chocolate doughs, appear much more complicated to make than they really are. And they taste as good as they look, especially served next to Tofu Ice Cream with Soy Chocolate Sauce (page 209) or Tofu Peach Whip (page 203).

Vanilla Cookie Dough

½ cup soy margarine

½ cup sugar

1½ cups unbleached all-purpose
   flour

1½ teaspoons baking powder

⅛ teaspoon salt

6 tablespoons soy milk

½ teaspoon vanilla extract

Chocolate Dough

½ cup soy margarine

½ cup sugar

1 cup unbleached all-purpose flour

1½ teaspoons baking powder

⅛ teaspoon salt

½ cup unsweetened cocoa powder

6 tablespoons soy milk

½ teaspoon vanilla extract

1. Make the vanilla dough and chocolate dough one at a time. For each, in a large mixing bowl, combine the soy margarine and sugar, and beat with a hand mixer until creamy.

2. In a medium bowl, mix the flour, baking powder, and salt. When making the chocolate dough, add the cocoa.

3. In a small bowl, combine the soy milk and vanilla.

4. Add the dry ingredients to the sugar and margarine mixture, alternating with milk and vanilla mixture until thoroughly mixed. The dough will be very stiff.

5. Roll dough out onto a lightly floured surface, and form into 2 rectangular logs, each 1½ inches thick and 8 inches long. Wrap the formed doughs in plastic or waxed paper, and refrigerate for 3 hours, or up to 3 days. (Dough can also be frozen up to 3 months.)

6. Unwrap the chilled vanilla and chocolate doughs and cut lenthwise into quarters.

7. Preheat the oven to 350°F., and line 2 cookie sheets with parchment paper.

8. Assemble the logs into 1 big log, using 2 sticks of chocolate and 2 of vanilla. Form a checkerboard pattern, pressing the pieces together gently to

avoid air pockets. Cut the log crosswise into ¼-inch slices and place each slice 1 inch apart on the cookie sheets.

9. Bake for 12 to 15 minutes on upper oven rack. Cool completely and store in airtight containers.

MAKES 72 COOKIES

Calories	Total Protein	Soy Protein	Carbohydrate	Fat	Cholesterol	Fiber	Sodium
51	1 g	0.5 g	6 g	2.7 g	0 mg	0 g	23 mg

Information is for 1 cookie.

Variation: To produce colored cookies for special occasions, add desired food coloring to vanilla dough in step 3.

Tofu Chocolate Mousse

The consistency of this silky dessert is indistinguishable from the richest, creamiest traditional chocolate mousse. This is the perfect way to end a meal—a chocolate treat that's good for you. It's also a great way to sneak tofu into your family's desserts. Chocolate pudding fans will never know the difference.

> 1 pound firm, silken tofu
> 1 cup honey
> ¾ cup unsweetened cocoa powder
> ½ teaspoon vanilla extract
> ½ cup raspberries, for garnish

1. In a food processor or blender, whip the tofu until smooth. Add the honey, cocoa, and vanilla and blend until well combined. Transfer to a serving bowl or divide among 6 parfait glasses and chill for 2 hours or overnight.

2. At serving time, garnish with raspberries and serve immediately.

SERVES 6

Calories	Total Protein	Soy Protein	Carbohydrate	Fat	Cholesterol	Fiber	Sodium
312	14 g	11 g	57 g	8 g	0 mg	1 g	22 mg

Information is per serving.

Cookie doughs made with soy are easy to double and they freeze beautifully. A time-saving tip is to make a double batch and wrap the extra dough tightly in plastic wrap. Store in the freezer for up to three months. That way, you'll be able to whip up homemade cookies on a moment's notice.

Alternatively, bake up a double batch of cookies and freeze the extras in airtight containers. All the cookies and biscotti in the book, as well as the brownies, will keep perfectly in the freezer for up to three months.

Chocolate Sandwich Cookies with Strawberry Soy Cream Cheese Filling

Think of these as Oreos for grown-ups. When you unscrew the rich, chocolatety top of this giant sandwich cookie, you'll find a delectable strawberry cream filling to lick off. Or fill the cookies with Tofu Ice Cream with Soy Chocolate Sauce (page 209) for sensational homemade ice cream sandwiches.

½ cup honey

⅓ cup plain soy yogurt

⅓ cup soy milk

¾ cup unsweetened cocoa powder

2¼ cups whole wheat pastry flour

¼ teaspoon baking soda

¾ cup (6 ounces) soy cream cheese

6 tablespoons (⅓ cup) strawberry
  preserves

1. Preheat the oven to 350°F. Line 2 cookie sheets with parchment paper.

2. In a food processor or blender, cream the honey, soy yogurt, and soy milk until smooth.

3. In a large bowl, sift together the cocoa powder, flour, and baking soda. Gradually add the yogurt mixture to the dry ingredients. The dough will be stiff.

4. On a floured surface, roll out the dough to a ¼-inch thickness and cut with a 3-inch cookie cutter.

5. Bake for 15 minutes, until cookies are firm. Remove from oven and cool completely.

6. While the cookies are cooling, blend the soy cream cheese and strawberry preserves. Spread the mixture between 2 chocolate cookies for each sandwich.

MAKES 8 VERY BIG SANDWICH COOKIES

Calories	Total Protein	Soy Protein	Carbohydrate	Fat	Cholesterol	Fiber	Sodium
293	8 g	3.6 g	47 g	9 g	0 mg	5 g	98 mg

Information is for 1 cookie.

Variation: To make delicious ice cream sandwiches, replace the strawberry filling with ½ cup of Tofu Ice Cream for each serving. Press down evenly on the cookies to distribute the ice cream and keep in the freezer until ready to serve.

Orange-Walnut Biscotti

It's okay to dunk biscotti: these hard, twice-baked Italian cookies were invented to be dipped in coffee or sweet dessert wines. They're also great on their own. Tofu replaces the eggs and butter here, but you'll never know the difference. Tangy orange zest balances the richness of the walnuts, a typical ingredient in Italian biscotti. These keep well in airtight tins for two weeks.

1 cup sugar	2 teaspoons vanilla extract
12 ounces soft tofu	3½ cups unbleached all-purpose
Zest from 1 medium orange,	flour
minced	2 teaspoons baking powder
2 tablespoons vegetable oil	¾ cup chopped walnuts

1. Blend the sugar and tofu in a food processor or blender until smooth.

2. Add the orange zest, oil, and vanilla, and process until blended.

3. In a large bowl, mix the flour, baking powder, and walnuts. Gradually add the tofu mixture, stirring with a wooden spoon until completely combined. Cover and chill for 30 minutes.

4. Preheat the oven to 325°F. and grease 2 cookie sheets or line with parchment paper.

5. Roll dough out onto a lightly floured surface, cut into quarters, and form each quarter into a log about 8 inches long.

6. Place the logs on the prepared cookie sheets and bake for 30 minutes, until dough is firm but not browned. Remove from oven.

7. Lower the oven temperature to 250°F. With a serrated knife, cut each log into 16 slices and return to the oven for 20 more minutes, until cookies are brown and hardened.

MAKES 64 BISCOTTI

Calories	Total Protein	Soy Protein	Carbohydrate	Fat	Cholesterol	Fiber	Sodium
53	1.5 g	0.6 g	8.6 g	1.5 g	0 mg	0.3 g	10 mg

Information is for 1 biscotto.

Tofu Chocolate Hazelnut Biscotti

Ground hazelnuts take the place of some of the flour in these dark chocolate biscotti, making them dense and rich. Serve with raspberry sorbet and a cup of good coffee.

1 cup sugar
12 ounces soft tofu
2 tablespoons vegetable oil
2 teaspoons vanilla extract
3 cups unbleached all-purpose flour
2 teaspoons baking powder
½ cup unsweetened cocoa powder
½ cup ground hazelnuts

1. Blend the sugar and tofu in a food processor or blender until smooth.
2. Add the oil and vanilla, and process until blended.
3. In a large bowl, mix the flour, baking powder, cocoa, and hazelnuts. With a wooden spoon, gradually mix in the tofu mixture until completely combined. Cover and chill for 30 minutes.
4. Preheat the oven to 325°F. and grease 2 cookie sheets or line with parchment paper.
5. Roll dough out onto a lightly floured surface, cut into quarters, and form each quarter into a log about 8 inches long.
6. Place the logs on the prepared cookie sheets and bake for 30 minutes, until dough is firm but not browned. Remove from oven.
7. Lower the oven temperature to 250°F. With a serrated knife, cut each log into 16 slices and return to the oven for 20 more minutes, until cookies are brown and hardened.

MAKES 64 BISCOTTI

Calories	Total Protein	Soy Protein	Carbohydrate	Fat	Cholesterol	Fiber	Sodium
52	1.5 g	0.6 g	8.6 g	1.5 g	0 mg	0 g	11 mg

Information is for 1 biscotto.

Soy Cream Cheese Fruit Bars

Bar cookies are much quicker to whip up than drop cookies. Here, chewy oatmeal layers enclose a sweet, fruit-and-cream-cheese filling. You'll find that using soy nuts instead of regular nuts in baked goods gives the same toothsome crunch, but adds soy goodness as well.

> 1½ cups unbleached all-purpose flour
> ¼ cup soy flour
> ¾ cup brown sugar
> 1 teaspoon baking powder
> 1 cup soy margarine, chilled
> 1½ cups quick-cooking rolled oats (not instant)
> ½ cup chopped soy nuts or walnuts
> 12 ounces apricot, raspberry, or strawberry pie filling
> 16 ounces soy cream cheese

1. Preheat the oven to 325° F. and grease a 13 × 9-inch baking pan.
2. In a medium bowl, combine the flours, brown sugar, and baking powder.
3. Cut in the margarine until mixture resembles coarse crumbs. Add the oats and walnuts, and mix until crumbly.
4. In a medium bowl, mix the fruit filling with the soy cream cheese until combined.
5. Pat half the oatmeal mixture into the baking pan. Spread the fruit filling over it, and top with the remaining flour mixture.
6. Bake for 30 minutes, or until slightly browned on top. Cool the mixture in the pan, and cut into bars.

MAKES 36 BARS

Calories	Total Protein	Soy Protein	Carbohydrate	Fat	Cholesterol	Fiber	Sodium
170	3.5 g	3 g	15 g	10 g	14 mg	1.2 g	51 mg

Information is for 1 bar.

Chocolate Tofu Ganache

2 cups semisweet tofu
  chocolate chips
1 cup soy milk

1. In a double boiler set
over simmering water, gradually combine the choco-
late chips with the soy
milk, stirring constantly
until the mixture is
smooth. Watch carefully, as
there is a tendency for
lumps to form.
2. Remove from heat and
slowly and evenly pour
over the cake until it is covered. Let cool and serve.

MAKES 2 1/2 CUPS

Calories: 273, Total Protein: 3.5 g,	
Soy Protein: 3.5 g,	
Carbohydrate: 40 g, Fat: 12.5 g,	
Cholesterol: 0 mg, Fiber: 0 g,	
Sodium: 42 mg	

Information is for 1/3 cup sauce.

Yellow Cake with Chocolate Tofu Ganache

The addition of soft tofu makes this cake moist and delicious. In this recipe, it's filled with strawberry jam and encased in smooth chocolate ganache, but you can use any filling or frosting you want. Ganache made with soy milk is less firm and glossy than standard ganache, which is made with heavy cream, but it is delicious nonetheless. I've included a simple fluffy chocolate cream cheese icing as a variation.

2¼ cups sifted cake flour
2 teaspoons baking powder
½ teaspoon salt
1¼ cups sugar
½ cup soy margarine
8 ounces soft tofu

1½ cups soy milk
2 teaspoons vanilla extract
½ cup strawberry jam
Chocolate Tofu Ganache (see
  sidebar)

1. Preheat the oven to 350° F. and grease and flour two 8 × 8-inch cake pans.
2. In a large bowl, combine the flour, baking powder, and salt and set aside.
3. With an electric mixer, beat the sugar and margarine together until creamy.
4. In a food processor or blender, mix the tofu, soy milk, and vanilla until smooth. Combine the tofu mixture with sugar and margarine and mix completely.
5. Gradually add the liquid mixture to the dry ingredients, stirring until thoroughly combined.
6. Pour the batter into the greased pans and bake for 30 minutes, or until a wooden pick inserted into the center comes out clean.
7. Cool until cakes reach room temperature. Spread strawberry jam evenly on one layer. Place the other layer on top. Coat with the ganache.

SERVES 8

Calories	Total Protein	Soy Protein	Carbohydrate	Fat	Cholesterol	Fiber	Sodium
390	6 g	3.5 g	61 g	13 g	0 mg	1 g	245 mg

Information is per serving.

Variation: For chocolate cream cheese frosting, combine 3 ounces softened soy cream cheese and ¼ cup soy milk. Gradually beat in 4 cups of confectioners' sugar and ½ teaspoon salt. Add 3 ounces melted chocolate and beat until smooth and fluffy.

Tofu Cheesecake

Take a traditional cheesecake recipe and replace the sour cream and cream cheese with soy equivalents. The result is amazingly similar to the original: dense, moist, and rich. If you're longing for chocolate cheesecake, simply add to this recipe ½ cup unsweetened cocoa and an extra ¼ cup of sugar.

> 1½ pounds silken tofu
>
> 1 cup sugar
>
> 12 ounces soy cream cheese
>
> 1 tablespoon vanilla extract
>
> 1 Graham Cracker Pie Crust (see sidebar)
>
> 1 cup (per cake) fresh berries, any kind (optional)

1. Have all the ingredients at room temperature. Preheat the oven to 325°F.

2. In a food processor or blender, puree the tofu until smooth. Add the sugar, soy cream cheese, and vanilla, processing until smooth. Scrape down the sides as necessary.

3. Pour the tofu mixture into prepared pie crust and bake for 50 minutes, until slightly browned.

4. Turn the oven off, leaving the cake in the oven for 1 hour. Remove and cool to room temperature.

5. Refrigerate the cheesecake overnight. Serve slightly chilled, garnished with fresh berries.

MAKES 2 9-INCH CHEESECAKES

Calories	Total Protein	Soy Protein	Carbohydrate	Fat	Cholesterol	Fiber	Sodium
268	6.5 g	5 g	27 g	14.5 g	0 mg	1 g	135 mg

Information is for ⅛ cheesecake, including berries.

Graham Cracker Pie Crust

2 cups graham crackers crumbs (about 16 whole crackers)

6 tablespoons soy margarine, slightly softened

1. Process the graham crackers in a food processor or blender on high speed until they are finely ground.

2. Add the margarine and pulse until the mixture reaches the consistency of coarse crumbs.

3. Pat the mixture into a thick layer in the bottom of an 8-inch springform pan, or 2 thinner layers in 9-inch pie plates. Fill and bake according to recipe instructions.

MAKES 1 8-INCH PIE CRUST

Pumpkin Tofu Cheesecake

I created this delectable dessert so I could indulge in two of my favorite sweets at once: cinnamony pumpkin pie and dense, rich cheesecake. Tradition with a twist, this makes a perfect holiday finale. But you don't have to wait for Thanksgiving.

1½ pounds silken tofu

1 cup canned or fresh cooked pumpkin

1¼ cups sugar

1 teaspoon ground cinnamon

½ teaspoon ground nutmeg

¼ teaspoon ground cloves

12 ounces soy cream cheese

1 tablespoon vanilla extract

2 9-inch Graham Cracker Pie Crusts (page 197)

1. Have all the ingredients at room temperature. Preheat the oven to 325°F.

2. In a food processor or blender, puree the tofu and pumpkin until smooth. Add the sugar, spices, soy cream cheese, and vanilla, processing until smooth. Scrape down the sides as necessary.

3. Pour the tofu mixture into prepared pie crusts and bake for 50 minutes, until the cheesecake mixture is firm.

4. Turn the oven off, leaving the cake in the oven for 1 hour. Remove and cool to room temperature.

5. Refrigerate the cheesecake overnight. Serve cool.

MAKES 2 9-INCH CHEESECAKES

Calories	Total Protein	Soy Protein	Carbohydrate	Fat	Cholesterol	Fiber	Sodium
268	5.5 g	4.5 g	28 g	14.5 g	0 mg	1.2 g	136 mg

Information is for ⅛ cheesecake.

Chocolate Tofu Almond Pie

You can make this scrumptious pie in minutes—and that's about as long as it will last when you serve it. This dessert, which is like a firm, dark chocolate pudding in a graham-cracker crust, is guaranteed to become a family favorite.

¾ cup slivered almonds

1 pound firm, silken tofu

1 cup brown sugar, tightly packed

1 cup unsweetened cocoa powder

1 teaspoon almond extract

1 9-inch Graham Cracker Pie Crust (page 197)

1. Preheat the oven to 350°F. Spread the slivered almonds on a baking sheet and place in the oven. Toast them for 5 to 10 minutes, until they color lightly, shaking the pan and watching them carefully so that they don't burn. Set aside to cool.

2. In a food processor or blender on high speed, puree the tofu until smooth. Add the brown sugar and blend until thoroughly combined.

3. Add the cocoa and vanilla and continue to blend until the mixture is smooth. Scrape down the sides of the blender if necessary. Pour the mixture into the crust and sprinkle the almond slivers evenly on top. Cover and chill for at least 2 hours or up to 24.

MAKES 1 9-INCH PIE

Calories	Total Protein	Soy Protein	Carbohydrate	Fat	Cholesterol	Fiber	Sodium
308.5	13.6 g	9 g	47 g	16 g	0 mg	2 g	136 mg

Information is for ⅛ pie.

Baking Temperatures for Soy Cream Cheese

An oven thermometer is an indispensable tool for a baker, especially if you're baking with soy cream cheese. Soy cheesecakes should be baked at 325°F., slightly lower than their dairy counterparts. If the oven is much hotter than that, the soy cream cheese will separate.

Tofu Lemon Coconut Pie

A take-off on rich coconut cream pie, this tropical treat replaces eggs with tofu. The result is a little denser, but creamy and every bit as delicious. A slice of this pie— with 13.5 grams of soy protein—satisfies your sweet tooth as well as your conscience.

1½ pounds firm, silken tofu
Juice and zest of 1 small lemon
½ cup brown sugar, tightly packed
¼ cup shredded unsweetened coconut, regular or low-fat
1 9-inch Graham Cracker Pie Crust (page 197)
Thin lemon slices, for garnish

1. In a food processor or blender on medium speed, puree the tofu until smooth. Add the lemon juice and brown sugar and continue blending until thoroughly combined. Scrape down the sides of the blender if necessary.
2. Turn the blender on high and add the lemon zest and shredded coconut. Blend for 10 seconds.
3. Pour the mixture into the crust and refrigerate, covered, for 2 hours or overnight. Serve chilled, garnished with lemon slices.

MAKES 1 9-INCH PIE

Calories	Total Protein	Soy Protein	Carbohydrate	Fat	Cholesterol	Fiber	Sodium
227.5	14 g	13.5 g	30 g	13 g	0 mg	1.6 g	135 mg

Information is for ⅛ pie.

Tofu Pumpkin Pie

The texture's the same; the flavor's the same: a spicy-sweet, silken-smooth holiday tradition. Tofu and pumpkin pie were meant for each other.

1 pound firm, silken tofu

1 cup soy sour cream

2 cups canned or cooked fresh pumpkin

1 cup brown sugar

1 teaspoon ground cinnamon

½ teaspoon ground ginger

¼ teaspoon ground nutmeg

¼ teaspoon ground cloves

1 9-inch Pie Crust (see sidebar)

1. Preheat the oven to 350°F.

2. Put the tofu and soy sour cream in the food processor or blender and puree until smooth. Add the pumpkin, brown sugar, and spices and continue to mix until all ingredients are thoroughly combined.

3. Pour the mixture into the crust and bake for 1 hour, until pumpkin pie mixture sets. Cool and serve warm or room temperature.

MAKES 1 9-INCH PIE

Calories	Total Protein	Soy Protein	Carbohydrate	Fat	Cholesterol	Fiber	Sodium
465	11.3 g	10 g	46 g	27 g	0 mg	3 g	321 mg

Information is for ⅛ pie.

Pie Crust

1⅔ cups all-purpose flour (whole wheat pastry flour may be used but the result will be a little heavier)

2 teapoons salt

1½ cups soy margarine, chilled

⅓ cup ice cold water

1. In a large mixing bowl, combine the flour and salt.

2. Add the margarine to the flour and salt. Using your fingers, work the ingredients together quickly until the mixture resembles coarse flakes.

3. Add the cold water gradually and mix until the dough holds together. Be careful not to overmix, or the crust will be tough. Gather it into a ball and flatten it out.

4. Cover dough with plastic wrap and refrigerate for at least 1 hour, or overnight.

5. Roll out dough to a ¼-inch thickness (divide the dough in half and roll out each to a ⅛-inch thickness). Let the dough rest in the refrigerator for 20 minutes. Line 2 8- or 9-inch pie plates with the dough, crimping the edges decoratively.

MAKES 2 8- OR 9-INCH CRUSTS

Calories: 199, Total Protein: 1.5 g,

Soy Protein: 0 g,

Carbohydrate: 98 g, Fat: 17 g,

Cholesterol: 0 mg, Fiber: 0 g,

Sodium: 273 mg

Information is for 2 pie crusts.

Peaches and Cream Brûlée

Take the sweetest summer peaches you can find, slice them into individual home-made graham-cracker crusts, sprinkle with blueberries and frost the fruit with lightly sweetened soy sour cream and brown sugar. Then caramelize the sugar under a hot broiler. This is a simple way to make the best of summer even better.

1 recipe for Graham Cracker Pie Crust (page 197)

2 cups soy sour cream

1 tablespoon granulated sugar

Zest of ½ lemon

3 ripe peaches, peeled and cubed

1 cup fresh blueberries

¾ cup brown sugar

1. In 6 ovenproof cups or soufflé dishes, press down the graham cracker crumbs firmly with your finger to form a crust in the bottoms and as much up the sides of each cup as possible. Chill briefly.

2. Preheat the broiler. Put the soy sour cream, granulated sugar, and lemon zest into a food processor or blender and process until thoroughly combined.

3. Distribute the peaches and blueberries among the cups, and pour the sour cream mixture over them.

4. Sprinkle brown sugar on each portion. Set the cups on a cookie sheet and put under the broiler for 1 minute or until browned.

5. Remove from oven, and serve immediately.

SERVES 6

Calories	Total Protein	Soy Protein	Carbohydrate	Fat	Cholesterol	Fiber	Sodium
395	3.3 g	2.3 g	51 g	19 g	0 mg	2.5 g	155 mg

Information is for 1 brûlée.

Tofu Peach Whip

Simple and refreshing, this smooth treat is a wonderful conclusion to a summer meal. Naturally, in a recipe this simple, the peaches must be bursting with flavor. For pizazz, serve this beside Black and White Soy Cookies (page 190).

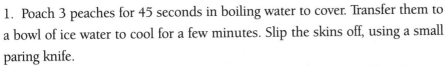

 4 ripe medium peaches
 1 pound silken, firm tofu
 ⅓ cup honey
 Mint sprigs, for garnish

1. Poach 3 peaches for 45 seconds in boiling water to cover. Transfer them to a bowl of ice water to cool for a few minutes. Slip the skins off, using a small paring knife.

2. Cut the peaches into slices and place in a food processor or blender. Add the tofu and honey and blend on high speed until the mixture is smooth, scraping down bowl as needed.

3. Divide the peach whip mixture among 6 dessert bowls and chill for 2 hours.

4. Peel the remaining peach and slice. Garnish each bowl with a peach slice and mint sprigs before serving.

SERVES 6

Calories	Total Protein	Soy Protein	Carbohydrate	Fat	Cholesterol	Fiber	Sodium
157	12 g	12 g	15 g	6 g	0 mg	2.5 g	11 mg

Information is per serving.

Variation: Substitute 1½ cups ripe strawberries for the 3 peaches. Garnish each serving with a whole strawberry.

Soy Tiramisù

In Italian, the word tiramisù *means "pick-me-up." This luscious layered dessert is so named because of the heady amount of strong, black coffee it contains. Crunchy tofu biscotti, dipped in coffee and coffee liqueur for flavor, line a bowl heaped with rich, vanilla cream cheese filling, topped with a dusting of cocoa powder. This will rate high on everyone's list of favorite desserts—and high as a source of soy protein, too. Hint: if you don't have time to make the biscotti, you can substitute store-bought ladyfingers, toasted briefly.*

16 ounces silken, firm tofu

2 tablespoons sugar

2 teaspoons vanilla extract

24 ounces soy cream cheese

2 cups strong black coffee

2 tablespoon coffee liqueur

24 Tofu Chocolate Hazelnut Biscotti (page 194)

3 tablespoons unsweetened cocoa powder

1. In a food processor or blender, combine the tofu, sugar, and vanilla and process until creamy.

2. Gradually add the soy cream cheese, pulsing after each addition until mixture is smooth.

3. In a small bowl, combine the coffee and coffee liqueur. Dip the biscotti quickly into the coffee mixture, moistening but not saturating them. They should hold their shape.

4. Place 2 biscotti in the bottom of an individual dessert bowl and cover with a layer of the tofu cheese mixture, another 2 biscotti, and another layer of tofu cheese mixture. Repeat the procedure in 5 more dessert bowls.

5. Refrigerate for 3 hours and dust with cocoa powder before serving.

SERVES 6

Calories	Total Protein	Soy Protein	Carbohydrate	Fat	Cholesterol	Fiber	Sodium
478	21.5 g	21 g	13 g	39.5 g	0 mg	1 g	364 mg

Information is per serving.

Tofu Flan

Tofu is a natural substitute for the eggs in flan, a Spanish dessert of smooth vanilla custard served with caramel syrup. The taste and consistency of this soy version is almost indistinguishable from the original.

12 ounces silken, firm tofu

6 ounces soy cream cheese

¼ cup soy milk

2 teaspoons vanilla extract

¼ cup honey

6 teaspoons brown sugar

1. Preheat the oven to 350°F.

2. Put all the ingredients except the brown sugar into a food processor or blender and mix until completely smooth.

3. Divide evenly among 6 custard dishes and bake for 15 minutes, until firm.

4. After 15 minutes, sprinkle 1 teaspoon of brown sugar on each custard dish. Continue baking for 5 more minutes, or until the tops have browned.

5. The flans can be served warm if desired, but the consistency improves with chilling. Let cool to room temperature before refrigerating for at least an hour.

SERVES 6

Calories	Total Protein	Soy Protein	Carbohydrate	Fat	Cholesterol	Fiber	Sodium
250	11 g	11 g	19.5 g	15 g	0 mg	0.8 g	96 mg

Information is for 1 flan.

Soy Dessert Crepes

Crepes are delicious, thin French pancakes used to enclose savory or sweet fillings or sauces. This basic batter recipe, which has sugar in it, is the one to use when you're making desserts. Some simple, yummy crepe desserts follow this recipe, and it's easy to come up with winners of your own—try filling crepes with strawberries and whipped cream or cooked apple slices, topped with caramel sauce. Crepes can be made ahead and frozen, wrapped in plastic with waxed paper or parchment between each one. Thaw them for an hour at room temperature before using in a recipe.

2 cups whole wheat flour
¼ cup sugar
2 tablespoons egg replacer
1 cup water

2 cups soy milk
2 tablespoons vegetable oil, plus a
    little for greasing pan

1. Measure the flour and sugar into a bowl and set aside.
2. In a food processor or blender, combine the egg replacer and water and blend until well mixed. Add the soy milk and oil and process briefly until thoroughly combined.
3. Add the flour mixture a cup at a time, pulsing between additions until smooth.
4. Place a crepe pan or small omelet pan over medium heat. Lightly brush the entire surface of the pan with oil. Lower the heat, leaving pan on low heat for about 3 minutes.
5. Lift the pan off the heat and pour in ¼ cup of the batter. Quickly tilt the pan in all directions, coating the bottom with a thin, even film of batter. Return the pan to the heat and cook until the crepe bubbles, about 45 seconds. Turn the crepe and cook the other side for about 30 seconds.
6. Stack the crepes on a plate for filling.

MAKES ABOUT 16

Calories	Total Protein	Soy Protein	Carbohydrate	Fat	Cholesterol	Fiber	Sodium
88	2 g	1 g	14 g	2 g	0 mg	0 g	4 mg

Information is for 1 crepe.

Orange Marmalade Crepes

You'll love this different approach to crepes—they're folded and coated with orange sauce, made from fresh oranges and tangy peel. It's simpler than filling and rolling crepes, and the flavor is fabulous. The citrus zing of this dessert makes it the perfect finishing touch to a meal of hearty stew or chili.

> 1 medium orange
> 4 tablespoons soy margarine
> 2 tablespoons sugar
> 1 cup orange juice
> 12 Soy Dessert Crepes (page 206)

1. Scrub the orange and cut it into thin slices. Cut each slice into quarters. Set aside.

2. In a saucepan over medium heat, melt the soy margarine. Add the sugar and orange juice, stirring until sugar is melted.

3. Add the orange slices and simmer over medium-low heat until the peel is tender.

4. Fold the crepes into quarters, place in a shallow serving dish, and spoon sauce over crepes. Serve warm.

SERVES 6

Calories	Total Protein	Soy Protein	Carbohydrate	Fat	Cholesterol	Fiber	Sodium
243	5 g	4 g	39 g	7 g	0 mg	2 g	10 mg

Information is for 2 crepes.

Dalmation Dessert Crepes

Dark mocha chips fleck the rich cream cheese filling in this incredible—and incredibly easy—dessert. The pancakes can be made ahead and frozen, in which case you can assemble this dessert in a matter of minutes. The coffee-chocolate flavor of the chips is my favorite, but you can substitute regular tofu chocolate chips, if desired. They're both available in health food stores and will satisfy any chocoholic.

24 ounces soy cream cheese

½ cup granulated sugar

2 teaspoons vanilla extract

⅓ cup tofu espresso chocolate chips or regular tofu chocolate chips

12 Soy Dessert Crepes (page 206)

3 tablespoons confectioners' sugar

1. Combine the cream cheese, granulated sugar, and vanilla in a large bowl, mixing well. Fold in the tofu-chocolate chips.
2. Fill each crepe with 3 tablespoons filling.
3. Roll the crepes into cylinders, place 2 on each plate, and dust with confectioners' sugar.

SERVES 6

Calories	Total Protein	Soy Protein	Carbohydrate	Fat	Cholesterol	Fiber	Sodium
600	9 g	4 g	54 g	14 g	0 mg	1 g	148 mg

Information is for 2 crepes.

Tofu Ice Cream with Soy Chocolate Sauce

Can a dessert this scrumptious still be good for you? Yes, when both the ice cream and the chocolate sauce contain such hefty doses of soy. This dark chocolate sauce glazes a silky-smooth, frozen tofu treat, and you'll think you're eating a hot-fudge sundae from the ice cream parlor. The chocolate sauce is great warm or cool.

> 2 pounds firm, silken tofu
> 1½ cups low-fat vanilla soy milk
> 6 tablespoons honey

1. In a food processor or blender, process all the ingredients until smooth.
2. Pour into an ice cream maker and freeze according to manufacturer's instructions. (The ice cream can be made up to 3 days ahead.)

SERVES 6

Calories	Total Protein	Soy Protein	Carbohydrate	Fat	Cholesterol	Fiber	Sodium
102	13 g	13 g	4 g	4 g	0 mg	2 g	18 mg

Information is for a ⅔-cup serving.

Variation: When you have crepes in the freezer, it is a snap to assemble another fabulous ice cream dessert. Spoon about ¼ cup of Tofu Ice Cream on each crepe, fold in half, and drizzle Soy Chocolate Sauce on top.

Soy Chocolate Sauce

4 ounces soft tofu
1½ cups soy milk
1 cup unsweetened cocoa powder
⅓ cup honey
1 teaspoon Kahlua, Amaretto, or orange extract (optional)

1. Combine all the ingredients in a food processor or blender and mix on high speed until completely pureed.
2. Serve at room temperature, warm, or chilled. Can be stored in refrigerator for up to 2 weeks.

MAKES ABOUT 3 CUPS

Calories: 30, Total Protein: 1.5 g,
Soy Protein: 0.5 g, Carbohydrate: 6 g,
Fat: 10 g, Cholesterol: 0 mg,
Fiber: 0 g, Sodium: 5 mg

Information is for a 1-ounce serving.

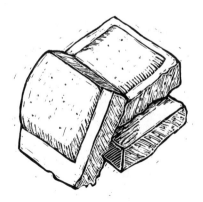

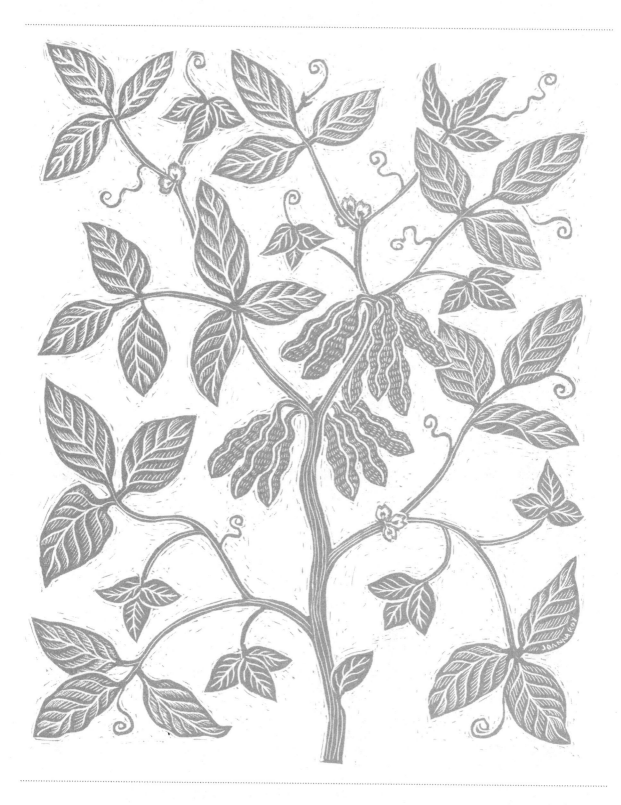

sources for soy products

Soy foods are becoming more and more widely distributed these days. Soy milk, soy cheeses, tofu, and soy meats once available only in health food stores can now be found in many ordinary grocery stores. Look for other products, such as tempeh, whole soybeans, and soy flour in health or specialty markets. If, however, you are having trouble locating certain products, call or write the following sources for direction to the nearest distributor. They may also be able to fill your needs by mail order.

Arrowhead Mills, Inc.
P.O. Box 2059
Hereford, Texas 79045
(800) 749-0730
(dried soybeans and flours)

Cloud Nine, Inc.
300 Observer Highway, Third Floor
Hoboken, New Jersey 07030
(201) 216-0382
(tofu chocolate chips)

Eden Foods, Inc.
701 Tecumseh Road
Clinton, Michigan 49236
(517) 456-7424
(soy milk)

Galaxy Foods, Soymage Products
2441 Viscount Row
Orlando, Florida 32809
(407) 855-5500/fax (407) 855-7485
(soy cheese, parmesan, cream cheese, sour cream)

Lisanatti Soy-Sation
P.J. Lisac and Associates
9001 S.E. Lawnfield Road
Clackamas, Oregon 97015
(503) 652-1988
(soy and nut-based cheese products)

LiteLife Foods, Inc.
P.O. Box 870
Greenfield, Massachusetts 01302
(800) 274-6001
(Gimme Lean soy sausage, soy Italian links, soy bacon, ham, soy pepperoni, and tempeh)

Mori Nu Tofu
2050 W. 190th Street, Suite 110
Torrance, California 90504
(800) 669-8638
(specially sealed 12.3-ounce packages of tofu)

Nasoya Foods, Inc.
23 Jytek Park
Leominster, Massachusetts 01453
(800) 229-8638
(soy mayonnaise)

SoyaKaas Cheeses, American Natural Snacks
P.O. Box 1067
St. Augustine, Florida 32085
(800) 238-3947
(soy cheese, parmesan, cream cheese)

Sweet Nothings, a division of Turtle Mountain, Inc.
P.O. Box 70
Junction City, Oregon 97448
(541) 998-6778
(It's Soy! frozen desserts)

Tofutti Brands, Inc.
50 Jackson Drive
Cranford, New Jersey 07016
(908) 272-2400/fax (908) 272-9492
(soy cream cheese, sour cream, filled pastas, frozen desserts, cookies)

Westbrae Natural Foods
1065 E. Walnut Street
Carson, California 90746
(800) 776-1276
(soy milk, canned soybeans)

White Wave, Inc.
1990 N. 57th Court
Boulder, Colorado 80301
(303) 443-3470
(soy yogurt, tofu, tempeh)

**Worthington Foods, Inc./
  Morningstar Farms**
900 Proprietors Road
Worthington, Ohio 43085-3194
(800) 243-1810
(ground soy sausage, soy burgers,
  soy bacon)

Yves Fine Foods
1638 Derwent Way
Delta, British Columbia V3M6R9
(800) 667-9837
(soy bacon, pepperoni, soy dogs,
  soy burgers)

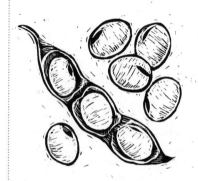

general information on soy

For more information about soy—its medical and health benefits and how to use it—call or write these knowledgeable sources:

American Soybean Association
540 Maryville Centre Drive,
   Suite 390
St. Louis, Missouri 63141
(314) 576-1770
(free recipes and information on
   soy products)

American Soybean Association
   Library-Archives
777 Craig Road
P.O. Box 27300
St. Louis, Missouri 63141
(314) 576-1770

Archer Daniels Midland (ADM)
   Corporation
Box 1470
Decatur, Illinois 62525
(800) 637-5850
(country's largest producer of soy
   products)

National Soybean Research
   Laboratory (NSRL)
University of Illinois at Urbana-
   Champaign
170 Environmental and
   Agricultural Sciences Building
1101 West Peabody Drive
Urbana, Illinois 61801
(217) 244-1706
(publishes a bulletin three times a
   year)

Ohio Soybean Council
Two Nationwide Plaza
P.O. Box 479
Columbus, Ohio 43216-1479
(614) 249-2492

Soyfoods Center
P.O. Box 234
Lafayette, California 94549
(510) 283-2991
(a resource center for information
   on soy and soy products)

United Soybean Hotline
6000 W. Executive Drive
P.O. Box 249
Mequon, Wisconsin 53092
(800) 825-5769
(soy recipes, health, and agricultural information)

index

about the author

Patricia Greenberg is a clinical dietician with a B.A. in nutrition and a graduate of the Scottsdale Culinary Institute. She operates a teaching consulting firm in Los Angeles called The Fitness Gourmet, which focuses on vegetarian and low-fat cooking classes locally and throughout the country. She is an expert in bringing a healthful approach to menu planning through plant-based organic foods, and has traveled extensively studying international cuisine. She lives in Los Angeles, California.

conversion chart

Equivalent Imperial and Metric Measurements

American cooks use standard containers, the 8-ounce cup and a tablespoon that takes exactly 16 level fillings to fill that cup level. Measuring by cup makes it very difficult to give weight equivalents, as a cup of densely packed butter will weigh considerably more than a cup of flour. The easiest way therefore to deal with cup measurements in recipes is to take the amount by volume rather than by weight. Thus the equation reads: 1 cup = 240 ml = 8 fl. oz.; ½ cup = 120 ml = 4 fl. oz. It is possible to buy a set of American cup measures in major stores around the world.

In the States, butter is often measured in sticks. One stick is the equivalent of 8 tablespoons. One tablespoon of butter is therefore the equivalent to ½ ounce/15 grams.

Liquid Measures

Fluid ounces	U.S.	Imperial	Milliliters
	1 teaspoon	1 teaspoon	5
¼	2 teaspoons	1 dessertspoon	10
½	1 tablespoon	1 tablespoon	14
1	2 tablespoons	2 tablespoons	28
2	¼ cup	4 tablespoons	56
4	½ cup or ¼ pint		110
5		¼ pint or 1 gill	140
6	¾ cup		170
8	1 cup or ½ pint		225
9			250, ¼ liter
10	1¼ cups	½ pint	280
12	1½ cups		340
15		¾ pint	420
16	2 cups or 1 pint		450
18	2¼ cups		500, ½ liter
20	2½ cups	1 pint	560
24	3 cups or 1½ pints		675
25		1¼ pints	700
27	3½ cups		750, ¾ liter
30	3¾ cups	1½ pints	840
32	4 cups or 2 pints or 1 quart		900

Solid Measures

U.S. and Imperial Measures		Metric Measures	
ounces	pounds	grams	kilos
1		28	
2		56	
3½		100	
4	¼	112	
5		140	
6		168	
8	½	225	
9		250	¼
12	¾	340	
16	1	450	
18		500	½
20	1¼	560	
24	1½	675	
27		750	¾
28	1¾	780	
32	2	900	
36	2¼	1000	1
40	2½	1100	
48	3	1350	
54		1500	1½
64	4	1800	
72	4½	2000	2

Equivalents for Ingredients

all-purpose flour—plain flour
arugula—rocket
confectioners' sugar—icing sugar
cornstarch—cornflour
eggplant—aubergine
granulated sugar—castor sugar
half-and-half—12% fat milk
lima beans—broad beans
scallion—spring onion
shortening—white fat
squash—courgettes or marrow
unbleached flour—strong, white flour
vanilla bean—vanilla pod
zest—rind
zucchini—courgettes

Oven Temperature Equivalents

Fahrenheit	Celsius	Gas Mark	Description
225	110	¼	Cool
250	130	½	
275	140	1	Very Slow
300	150	2	
325	170	3	Slow
350	180	4	Moderate
375	190	5	
400	200	6	Moderately Hot
425	220	7	Fairly Hot
450	230	8	Hot
475	240	9	Very Hot
500	250	10	Extremely Hot

Linear and Area Measures

1 inch	2.54 centimeters